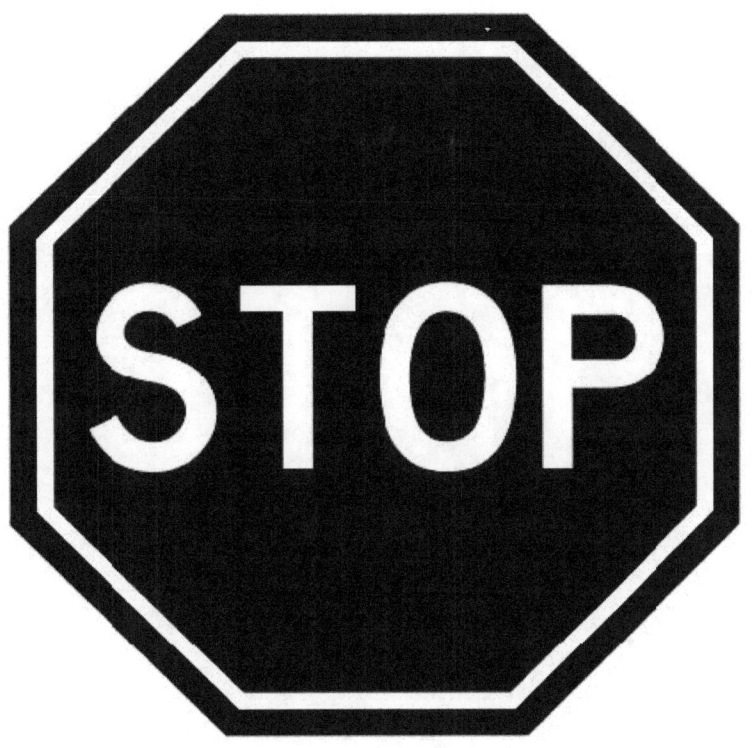

FREE Test Taking Tips DVD Offer

To help us better serve you, we have developed a Test Taking Tips DVD that we would like to give you for FREE. **This DVD covers world-class test taking tips that you can use to be even more successful when you are taking your test.**

All that we ask is that you email us your feedback about your study guide. Please let us know what you thought about it – whether that is good, bad or indifferent.

To get your **FREE Test Taking Tips DVD**, email freedvd@studyguideteam.com with "FREE DVD" in the subject line and the following information in the body of the email:

  a. The title of your study guide.

  b. Your product rating on a scale of 1-5, with 5 being the highest rating.

  c. Your feedback about the study guide. What did you think of it?

  d. Your full name and shipping address to send your free DVD.

If you have any questions or concerns, please don't hesitate to contact us at freedvd@studyguideteam.com.

Thanks again!

PTCB Exam Study Guide

PTCE Exam Study Guide Team

Copyright © 2017 PTCE Exam Study Guide Team

All rights reserved.

Table of Contents

Quick Overview 1
Test-Taking Strategies 2
FREE DVD OFFER 6
Introduction to the Pharmacy Technician Certification Exam (PTCE) 7
Pharmacology for Technicians 9
    Practice Questions 46
    Answer Explanations 48
Pharmacy Law and Regulations 49
    Practice Questions 68
    Answer Explanations 70
Sterile & Non-Sterile Compounding 72
    Practice Questions 86
    Answer Explanations 88
Medication Safety 89
    Practice Questions 97
    Answer Explanations 100
Pharmacy Quality Assurance 104
    Practice Questions 110
    Answer Explanations 112
Medication Order Entry and Fill Process 114
    Practice Questions 139
    Answer Explanations 141
Pharmacy Inventory Management 143
    Practice Questions 156
    Answer Explanations 159
Pharmacy Billing and Reimbursement 161
    Practice Questions 169
    Answer Explanations 170
Information System Usage and Application 171
    Practice Questions 177
    Answer Explanations 178

Quick Overview

As you draw closer to taking your exam, effective preparation becomes more and more important. Thankfully, you have this study guide to help you get ready. Use this guide to help keep your studying on track and refer to it often.

This study guide contains several key sections that will help you be successful on your exam. The guide contains tips for what you should do the night before and the day of the test. Also included are test-taking tips. Knowing the right information is not always enough. Many well-prepared test takers struggle with exams. These tips will help equip you to accurately read, assess, and answer test questions.

A large part of the guide is devoted to showing you what content to expect on the exam and to helping you better understand that content. Near the end of this guide is a practice test so that you can see how well you have grasped the content. Then, answer explanations are provided so that you can understand why you missed certain questions.

Don't try to cram the night before you take your exam. This is not a wise strategy for a few reasons. First, your retention of the information will be low. Your time would be better used by reviewing information you already know rather than trying to learn a lot of new information. Second, you will likely become stressed as you try to gain a large amount of knowledge in a short amount of time. Third, you will be depriving yourself of sleep. So be sure to go to bed at a reasonable time the night before. Being well-rested helps you focus and remain calm.

Be sure to eat a substantial breakfast the morning of the exam. If you are taking the exam in the afternoon, be sure to have a good lunch as well. Being hungry is distracting and can make it difficult to focus. You have hopefully spent lots of time preparing for the exam. Don't let an empty stomach get in the way of success!

When travelling to the testing center, leave earlier than needed. That way, you have a buffer in case you experience any delays. This will help you remain calm and will keep you from missing your appointment time at the testing center.

Be sure to pace yourself during the exam. Don't try to rush through the exam. There is no need to risk performing poorly on the exam just so you can leave the testing center early. Allow yourself to use all of the allotted time if needed.

Remain positive while taking the exam even if you feel like you are performing poorly. Thinking about the content you should have mastered will not help you perform better on the exam.

Once the exam is complete, take some time to relax. Even if you feel that you need to take the exam again, you will be well served by some down time before you begin studying again. It's often easier to convince yourself to study if you know that it will come with a reward!

Test-Taking Strategies

1. Predicting the Answer

When you feel confident in your preparation for a multiple-choice test, try predicting the answer before reading the answer choices. This is especially useful on questions that test objective factual knowledge or that ask you to fill in a blank. By predicting the answer before reading the available choices, you eliminate the possibility that you will be distracted or led astray by an incorrect answer choice. You will feel more confident in your selection if you read the question, predict the answer, and then find your prediction among the answer choices. After using this strategy, be sure to still read all of the answer choices carefully and completely. If you feel unprepared, you should not attempt to predict the answers. This would be a waste of time and an opportunity for your mind to wander in the wrong direction.

2. Reading the Whole Question

Too often, test takers scan a multiple-choice question, recognize a few familiar words, and immediately jump to the answer choices. Test authors are aware of this common impatience, and they will sometimes prey upon it. For instance, a test author might subtly turn the question into a negative, or he or she might redirect the focus of the question right at the end. The only way to avoid falling into these traps is to read the entirety of the question carefully before reading the answer choices.

3. Looking for Wrong Answers

Long and complicated multiple-choice questions can be intimidating. One way to simplify a difficult multiple-choice question is to eliminate all of the answer choices that are clearly wrong. In most sets of answers, there will be at least one selection that can be dismissed right away. If the test is administered on paper, the test taker could draw a line through it to indicate that it may be ignored; otherwise, the test taker will have to perform this operation mentally or on scratch paper. In either case, once the obviously incorrect answers have been eliminated, the remaining choices may be considered. Sometimes identifying the clearly wrong answers will give the test taker some information about the correct answer. For instance, if one of the remaining answer choices is a direct opposite of one of the eliminated answer choices, it may well be the correct answer. The opposite of obviously wrong is obviously right! Of course, this is not always the case. Some answers are obviously incorrect simply because they are irrelevant to the question being asked. Still, identifying and eliminating some incorrect answer choices is a good way to simplify a multiple-choice question.

4. Don't Overanalyze

Anxious test takers often overanalyze questions. When you are nervous, your brain will often run wild, causing you to make associations and discover clues that don't actually exist. If you feel that this may be a problem for you, do whatever you can to slow down during the test. Try taking a deep breath or counting to ten. As you read and consider the question, restrict yourself to the particular words used by the author. Avoid thought tangents about what the author *really* meant, or what he or she was *trying* to say. The only things that matter on a multiple-choice test are the words that are actually in the question. You must avoid reading too much into a multiple-choice question, or supposing that the writer meant something other than what he or she wrote.

5. No Need for Panic

It is wise to learn as many strategies as possible before taking a multiple-choice test, but it is likely that you will come across a few questions for which you simply don't know the answer. In this situation, avoid panicking. Because most multiple-choice tests include dozens of questions, the relative value of a single wrong answer is small. Moreover, your failure on one question has no effect on your success elsewhere on the test. As much as possible, you should compartmentalize each question on a multiple-choice test. In other words, you should not allow your feelings about one question to affect your success on the others. When you find a question that you either don't understand or don't know how to answer, just take a deep breath and do your best. Read the entire question slowly and carefully. Try rephrasing the question a couple of different ways. Then, read all of the answer choices carefully. After eliminating obviously wrong answers, make a selection and move on to the next question.

6. Confusing Answer Choices

When working on a difficult multiple-choice question, there may be a tendency to focus on the answer choices that are the easiest to understand. Many people, whether consciously or not, gravitate to the answer choices that require the least concentration, knowledge, and memory. This is a mistake. When you come across an answer choice that is confusing, you should give it extra attention. A question might be confusing because you do not know the subject matter to which it refers. If this is the case, don't eliminate the answer before you have affirmatively settled on another. When you come across an answer choice of this type, set it aside as you look at the remaining choices. If you can confidently assert that one of the other choices is correct, you can leave the confusing answer aside. Otherwise, you will need to take a moment to try to better understand the confusing answer choice. Rephrasing is one way to tease out the sense of a confusing answer choice.

7. Your First Instinct

Many people struggle with multiple-choice tests because they overthink the questions. If you have studied sufficiently for the test, you should be prepared to trust your first instinct once you have carefully and completely read the question and all of the answer choices. There is a great deal of research suggesting that the mind can come to the correct conclusion very quickly once it has obtained all of the relevant information. At times, it may seem to you as if your intuition is working faster even than your reasoning mind. This may in fact be true. The knowledge you obtain while studying may be retrieved from your subconscious before you have a chance to work out the associations that support it. Verify your instinct by working out the reasons that it should be trusted.

8. Key Words

Many test takers struggle with multiple-choice questions because they have poor reading comprehension skills. Quickly reading and understanding a multiple-choice question requires a mixture of skill and experience. To help with this, try jotting down a few key words and phrases on a piece of scrap paper. Doing this concentrates the process of reading and forces the mind to weigh the relative importance of the question's parts. In selecting words and phrases to write down, the test taker thinks about the question more deeply and carefully. This is especially true for multiple-choice questions that are preceded by a long prompt.

9. Subtle Negatives

One of the oldest tricks in the multiple-choice test writer's book is to subtly reverse the meaning of a question with a word like *not* or *except*. If you are not paying attention to each word in the question, you can easily be led astray by this trick. For instance, a common question format is, "Which of the following is…?" Obviously, if the question instead is, "Which of the following is not…?," then the answer will be quite different. Even worse, the test makers are aware of the potential for this mistake and will include one answer choice that would be correct if the question were not negated or reversed. A test taker who misses the reversal will find what he or she believes to be a correct answer and will be so confident that he or she will fail to reread the question and discover the original error. The only way to avoid this is to practice a wide variety of multiple-choice questions and to pay close attention to each and every word.

10. Reading Every Answer Choice

It may seem obvious, but you should always read every one of the answer choices! Too many test takers fall into the habit of scanning the question and assuming that they understand the question because they recognize a few key words. From there, they pick the first answer choice that answers the question they believe they have read. Test takers who read all of the answer choices might discover that one of the latter answer choices is actually *more* correct. Moreover, reading all of the answer choices can remind you of facts related to the question that can help you arrive at the correct answer. Sometimes, a misstatement or incorrect detail in one of the latter answer choices will trigger your memory of the subject and will enable you to find the right answer. Failing to read all of the answer choices is like not reading all of the items on a restaurant menu: you might miss out on the perfect choice.

11. Spot the Hedges

One of the keys to success on multiple-choice tests is paying close attention to every word. This is never more true than with words like *almost*, *most*, *some*, and *sometimes*. These words are called "hedges" because they indicate that a statement is not totally true or not true in every place and time. An absolute statement will contain no hedges, but in many subjects, like literature and history, the answers are not always straightforward or absolute. There are always exceptions to the rules in these subjects. For this reason, you should favor those multiple-choice questions that contain hedging language. The presence of qualifying words indicates that the author is taking special care with his or her words, which is certainly important when composing the right answer. After all, there are many ways to be wrong, but there is only one way to be right! For this reason, it is wise to avoid answers that are absolute when taking a multiple-choice test. An absolute answer is one that says things are either all one way or all another. They often include words like *every*, *always*, *best*, and *never*. If you are taking a multiple-choice test in a subject that doesn't lend itself to absolute answers, be on your guard if you see any of these words.

12. Long Answers

In many subject areas, the answers are not simple. As already mentioned, the right answer often requires hedges. Another common feature of the answers to a complex or subjective question are qualifying clauses, which are groups of words that subtly modify the meaning of the sentence. If the question or answer choice describes a rule to which there are exceptions or the subject matter is complicated, ambiguous, or confusing, the correct answer will require many words in order to be expressed clearly and accurately. In essence, you should not be deterred by answer choices that seem excessively long. Oftentimes, the author of the text will not be able to write the correct answer without offering some qualifications and modifications. Your job is to read the answer choices thoroughly and completely and to select the one that most accurately and precisely answers the question.

13. Restating to Understand

Sometimes, a question on a multiple-choice test is difficult not because of what it asks but because of how it is written. If this is the case, restate the question or answer choice in different words. This process serves a couple of important purposes. First, it forces you to concentrate on the core of the question. In order to rephrase the question accurately, you have to understand it well. Rephrasing the question will concentrate your mind on the key words and ideas. Second, it will present the information to your mind in a fresh way. This process may trigger your memory and render some useful scrap of information picked up while studying.

14. True Statements

Sometimes an answer choice will be true in itself, but it does not answer the question. This is one of the main reasons why it is essential to read the question carefully and completely before proceeding to the answer choices. Too often, test takers skip ahead to the answer choices and look for true statements. Having found one of these, they are content to select it without reference to the question above. Obviously, this provides an easy way for test makers to play tricks. The savvy test taker will always read the entire question before turning to the answer choices. Then, having settled on a correct answer choice, he or she will refer to the original question and ensure that the selected answer is relevant. The mistake of choosing a correct-but-irrelevant answer choice is especially common on questions related to specific pieces of objective knowledge, like historical or scientific facts. A prepared test taker will have a wealth of factual knowledge at his or her disposal, and should not be careless in its application.

15. No Patterns

One of the more dangerous ideas that circulates about multiple-choice tests is that the correct answers tend to fall into patterns. These erroneous ideas range from a belief that B and C are the most common right answers, to the idea that an unprepared test-taker should answer "A-B-A-C-A-D-A-B-A." It cannot be emphasized enough that pattern-seeking of this type is exactly the WRONG way to approach a multiple-choice test. To begin with, it is highly unlikely that the test maker will plot the correct answers according to some predetermined pattern. The questions are scrambled and delivered in a random order. Furthermore, even if the test maker was following a pattern in the assignation of correct answers, there is no reason why the test taker would know which pattern he or she was using. Any attempt to discern a pattern in the answer choices is a waste of time and a distraction from the real work of taking the test. A test taker would be much better served by extra preparation before the test than by reliance on a pattern in the answers.

FREE DVD OFFER

Don't forget that doing well on your exam includes both understanding the test content and understanding how to use what you know to do well on the test. We offer a completely FREE Test Taking Tips DVD that covers world class test taking tips that you can use to be even more successful when you are taking your test.

All that we ask is that you email us your feedback about your study guide. To get your **FREE Test Taking Tips DVD**, email freedvd@studyguideteam.com with "FREE DVD" in the subject line and the following information in the body of the email:

- The title of your study guide.
- Your product rating on a scale of 1-5, with 5 being the highest rating.
- Your feedback about the study guide. What did you think of it?
- Your full name and shipping address to send your free DVD.

Introduction to the Pharmacy Technician Certification Exam (PTCE)

Function of the Test

The Pharmacy Technician Certification Exam (PTCE) is administered by the Pharmacy Technician Certification Board (PTCB) and is used as part of the licensing process for Pharmacy Technicians. In many U.S. states. The PTCB reports that certified pharmacy technicians earn more money and have more access to promotions than those who are not certified. Test scores are typically used only in the certification process; employers do not typically request or consider the scores directly.

Most people taking the test are individuals looking to enhance their credentials to make progress in a career as a pharmacy technician. The test is administered nationwide, and states that use it are distributed around the country.

Test Administration

Test candidates must apply to take the PTCE and pay the test fee. Candidates whose applications are approved will receive an authorization at which time they will have ninety days to schedule their exam. The exam is given at any available time at Pearson VUE testing centers around the country.

Candidates are allowed up to four attempts to pass the PTCE. Candidates who do not pass must wait sixty days before a second or third attempt, and six months before a fourth attempt. After four attempts, interested individuals must submit a written request for additional attempts, which will be evaluated by the PTCB on a case-by-case basis. Such a request must spell out the specific steps that the candidate plans to take to obtain a successful result.

The PTCB will grant accommodations for students with disabilities, in cases where the requested accommodations are reasonable and consistent with the Americans with Disabilities Act (ADA).

Test Format

The PTCE consists of ninety questions, each with four multiple-choice answers. Ten of the ninety questions are unscored, although test takers do not know which ten. The test lasts 110 minutes, with another ten minutes set aside for a tutorial and post-exam survey. There are no breaks included in the testing time.

The test is administered on a computer. Test takers are not allowed to bring their own calculator, but they may request a calculator from the testing staff, and there is an on-screen calculator built into the testing program.

The content of the PTCE is divided between nine domains, which are as follows:

Domain	Percentage of Test
Pharmacology for Technicians	13.75%
Pharmacy Law and Regulations	12.5%
Sterile and Non-Sterile Compounding	8.75%
Medication Safety	12.5%
Pharmacy Quality Assurance	7.5%
Medication Order Entry and Fill Process	17.5%
Pharmacy Inventory Management	8.75%
Pharmacy Billing and Reimbursement	8.75%
Pharmacy Information Systems Usage and Application	10%

Scoring

Scores for the PTCE are based on the total number of correct answers given by the test taker. There is no penalty for incorrect answers or guesses and no benefit to leaving responses blank. The PTCB creates a reference score based off of an analysis of test items in which experts estimate the percentage of qualified pharmacy technicians that would be able to answer a given question. Those percentages are averaged together and scaled to a standard scale ranging from 1000 to 1600, with a passing score set at 1400. In 2015, 56,253 PTCEs were administered and with 31,823 passing marks achieved, for an overall passing rate of 57 percent.

Recent/Future Developments

The PTCE is updated approximately every five years, and the last update went into effect on November 1, 2013. At that time, score reports began reflecting scores for each of the nine domains, the scoring scale changed, and a new practice exam was published. A new update is due in 2018.

Pharmacology for Technicians

Generic and Brand Names of Pharmaceuticals

Generic drugs are subjected to a similar review process as brand-name drugs to ensure safety, efficacy, and quality. Generally, generic drugs are copies of the brand-name drug, and allow more affordable access to treatment and care. Pharmacy technicians should be familiar with the major therapeutic classifications of medications, and should be able to match brand names of medications with the corresponding generic names.

Drug Abbreviations

There are common abbreviations that are used for certain medications. The table below provides the abbreviations and the drug names for some of these medications:

Common Abbreviation	Medication
APAP	Acetaminophen
ASA	Aspirin
Fe	Iron
HCTZ	Hydrochlorothiazide
INH	Isoniazid
MgSO4	Magnesium sulfate
MOM	Milk of magnesia
MVI	Multivitamin
NS	Normal saline
NTG	Nitroglycerin
PCN	Penicillin
PNV	Prenatal vitamins
SMZ/TMP	Sulfamethoxazole/ trimethoprim
TAC	Triamcinolone
TCN	Tetracycline

Brand vs. Generic Names

Brand Name	Generic Name	Class of Medication (Treatment of)
Medications Acting on the Nervous System		
Dilantin®	Phenytoin	Anti-convulsant (seizure)
Keppra®	Levetiracetam	Anti-convulsant (seizure)
Depakote®	Divalproex	Anti-convulsant (seizure)
Celexa®	Citalopram	SSRI (anxiety and depression)
Lexapro®	Escitalopram	SSRI (anxiety and depression)
Prozac®	Fluoxetine	SSRI (anxiety and depression)
Paxil®	Paroxetine	SSRI (anxiety and depression)
Zoloft®	Sertraline	SSRI (anxiety and depression)
Effexor®	Venlafaxine	SNRI (anxiety and depression)
Cymbalta®	Duloxetine	SNRI (anxiety and depression)
Wellbutrin®	Bupropion	NDRI (anxiety and depression)
Seroquel®	Quetiapine	Anti-psychotic (Schizophrenia, bipolar disorder)
Risperdal®	Risperidone	Anti-psychotic (Schizophrenia, bipolar disorder)
Zyprexa®	Olanzapine	Anti-psychotic (Schizophrenia, bipolar disorder)
Abilify®	Aripiprazole	Anti-psychotic (Schizophrenia, bipolar disorder)
Geodon®	Ziprasidone	Anti-psychotic (Schizophrenia, bipolar disorder)
Topamax®	Topiramate	Anticonvulsant (seizure, migraine)
Tegretol®	Carbamazepine	Anticonvulsant (seizure)
Tileptal®	Oxcarbzepine	Anticonvulsant (seizure)
Depakote®	Valproic acid	Anticonvulsant (seizure)
Lamictal®	Lamotrigine	Anticonvulsant (seizure)
Keppra®	Levetiracetam	Anticonvulsant (seizure)
Dilantin®	Phenytoin	Anticonvulsant (seizure)
Neurontin®	Gabapentin	Anticonvulsant (seizure, neuropathic pain)
Lyrica®	Pregabalin	Anticonvulsant (seizure, neuropathic pain)
Aricept®	Donepezil	Cognition enhancer (Alzheimer disease
Namenda®	Memantine	Cognition enhancer (Alzheimer disease
Requip®	Ropinirole	Dopamine agonist (Parkinson's disease)
Mirapex®	Pramipexole	Dopamine agonist (Parkinson's disease)
Sinemet®	Levodopa & carbidopa	Dopamine agonist (Parkinson's disease)
Ambien®	Zolpidem	Sedative (insomnia)
Lunesta®	Eszopiclone	Sedative (insomnia)
Strattera®	Atomoxetine	Stimulant(ADHD)
Ritalin®	Methylphenidate	Stimulant (ADHD)
Adderall®	Mixed salt of amphetamine	Stimulants (ADHD)
Concerta®	Methylphenidate	Stimulants (ADHD)
Vyvanse®	Lisdexamfetamine	Stimulants (ADHD)
Provigil®	Modafinil	Stimulants (sleep disorder)
Maxalt®	Rizatriptan	Triptan (migraine)
Imitrex®	Sumatriptan	Triptan (migraine)
Medications Acting on the Cardiovascular System		
Zestril®	Lisinopril	ACE inhibitor (hypertension)
Zestoretic®	Lisinopril & HCTZ	ACE inhibitor & diuretic (hypertension)

Brand Name	Generic Name	Class of Medication (Treatment of)
Altace®	Ramipril	ACE inhibitor (hypertension)
Altace® HCT	Ramipril & HCTZ	ACE inhibitor & diuretic (hypertension)
Diovan®	Valsartan	ARB (hypertension)
Diovan® HCT	Valsartan & HCTZ	ARB & diuretic (hypertension)
Cozaar®	Losartan	ARB (hypertension)
Hyzaar®	Losartan & HCTZ	ARB & diuretic (hypertension)
Avapro®	Irbesartan	ARB (hypertension)
Avalide®	Irbesartan & HCTZ	ARB & diuretic (hypertension)
Atacand®	Candesartan	ARB (hypertension)
Atacand® Plus	Candesartan & HCTZ	ARB & diuretic (hypertension)
Micardis®	Telmisartan	ARB (hypertension)
Micardis® Plus	Telmisartan & HCTZ	ARB & diuretic (hypertension)
Benicar®	Olmesartan	ARB (hypertension)
Benicar® HCT	Olmesartan & HCTZ	ARB & diuretic (hypertension)
Inderal®	Propranolol	Beta-blocker (hypertension)
Toprol®	Metoprolol	Beta-blocker (hypertension)
Coreg®	Carvedilol	Beta-blocker (hypertension)
Norvasc®	Amlodipine	CCB (hypertension)
Lotrel®	Amlodipine & benazepril	CCB & ACEI (hypertension)
Zocor®	Simvastatin	Statin (hyperlipidemia)
Lipitor®	Atorvastatin	Statin (hyperlipidemia)
Crestor®	Rosuvastatin	Statin (hyperlipidemia)
Pravachol®	Pravastatin	Statin (hyperlipidemia)
Zetia®	Ezetimibe	Absorption inhibitor (hyperlipidemia)
Tricor®	Fenofibrate	Fibrate (hyperlipidemia)
Vytorin®	Ezetimibe & Simvastatin	Absorption inhibitor & statin (hyperlipidemia)
Plavix®	Clopidogrel	Blood thinner (blood clot)
Coumadin®	Warfarin	Blood thinner (blood clot)
Xarelto®	Rivaroxaban	Blood thinner (blood clot)
Eliquis®	Epixaban	Blood thinner (blood clot)
Lanoxin®	Digoxin	Glycoside (heart failure)
Digitek®	Digoxin	Glycoside (heart failure)
Klor-Con®	Potassium	Potassium supplement (hypokalemia)
Medications Acting on the Respiratory System		
Singulair	Montelukast	Anti-inflammatory (Asthma)
Nasonex®	Mometasone	Steroid (asthma, allergy)
Flovent®	Fluticasone	Steroid (asthma, COPD, allergy)
Ventolin®	Albuterol	Bronchodilator (Asthma
Combivent®	Albuterol/ipratropium	Bronchodilator (asthma, COPD)
Spiriva®	Tiotropium	Bronchodilator (COPD)
Rhinocort®	Budesonide	Steroid (nasal allergy)
Pulmicort®	Budesonide	Steroid (asthma, COPD)
Advair®	Fluticasone/salmeterol	Steroid/bronchodilatory (Asthma, COPD)
Symbicort®	Budesonide/formoterol	Steroid/bronchodilatory (Asthma, COPD)
Medications Acting on the Digestive System		
Prilosec®	Omeprazole	PPI (GERD)
Nexium®	Esomeprazole	PPI (GERD)

Brand Name	Generic Name	Class of Medication (Treatment of)
Prevacid®	Lansoprazole	PPI (GERD)
Protonix®	Pantoprazole	PPI (GERD)
AcipHex®	Rabeprazole	PPI (GERD)
Medications Acting on the Urinary System		
Flomax®	Tamsulosin	Urinary retainer (BPH)
Detrol®	Tolterodine	Bladder relaxant (urinary incontinence)
Viagra®	Sildenafil	Vasodilator (erectile dysfunction)
Cialis®	Tadalafil	Vasodilator (erectile dysfunction)
Levitra®	Vardenafil	Vasodilator (erectile dysfunction)
Medications Acting on the Endocrine System		
Glucophage®	Metformin	Anti-diabetic (type 2 diabetes)
Actos®	Pioglitazone	Anti-diabetic (type 2 diabetes)
Januvia®	Sitagliptin	Anti-diabetic (type 2 diabetes)
Janumet®	Sitagliptin/metformin	Anti-diabetic (type 2 diabetes)
Lantus®	insulin glargine	Anti-diabetic (type 1 and type 2 diabetes)
Humalog®	insulin lispro	Anti-diabetic (type 1 and type 2 diabetes)
Byetta®	Exenatide	Anti-diabetic (type 2 diabetes)
Synthroid®	Levothyroxine	Hormone (hypothryroidism)
Levoxyl®	Levothyroxine	Hormone (hypothryroidism)
Premarin®	conjugated estrogens	Hormone (postmenopausal symptoms)
Medications Acting on the Immune System		
Amoxil®	Amoxicillin	Antibiotic (infections)
Zithromax®	Azithromycin	Antibiotic (infections)
Levaquin®	Levofloxacin	Antibiotic (infections)
Omnicef®	Cefdinir	Antibiotic (infections)
Avelox®	Moxifloxacin	Antibiotic (infections)
Biaxin®	Clarithromycin	Antibiotic (infections)
Ciprodex®	Ciprofloxacin/dexamethasone	Antibiotic/steroid (ear infection)
TobraDex®	Tobramycin/dexamethasone	Antibiotic/steroid (eye infection)
Valtrex®	Valacyclovir	Anti-viral (herpes)
Viread®	Tenofovir	Anti-viral (hepatitis B, HIV)
Lamisil®	Terbinafine	Anti-fungal
Medications Acting on the Muscular and Skeletal System		
Fosamax®	Alendronate	Bone density modifier (osteoporosis)
Actonel®	Risedronate	Bone density modifier (osteoporosis)
Boniva®	Ibandronate	Bone density modifier (osteoporosis)
Evista®	Raloxifene	Estrogen modulator (osteoporosis)
Skelaxin®	Metaxalone	Muscle relaxant (musculoskeletal conditions)
Lidoderm®	Lidocaine	Anesthetic (pain)
Vicodin®	Hydrocodone/acetaminophen	Opioid/NSAID (pain)
Percocet®	Oxycodone/acetaminophen	Opioid/NSAID (pain)
Celebrex®	Celecoxib	NSAID (Pain)
Mobic®	Meloxicam	NSAID (Pain)
Medications Acting on the Eyes		
Xalatan®	Latanoprost	Anti-glaucoma (increased intraocular pressure)
Cosopt®	dorzolamide/timolol	Anti-glaucoma (increased intraocular pressure)
Lumigan®	Bimatoprost	Anti-glaucoma (increased intraocular pressure)

Brand Name	Generic Name	Class of Medication (Treatment of)
Travatan®	Travoprost	Anti-glaucoma (increased intraocular pressure)
Alphagan®	Brimonidine	Anti-glaucoma (increased intraocular pressure)
Zyrtec®	Cetirizine	Anti-histamine (allergy)
Allegra®	Fexofenadine	Anti-histamine (allergy)
Flonase®	Fluticasone	Anti-histamine (allergy)
Astelin®	Azelastine	Anti-histamine (allergy)
Patanol®	Olopatadine	Anti-histamine (eye allergies)

Abbreviation key: ADHD: attention-deficit hyperactivity disorder, ACEI: angiotensin converting enzyme inhibitor, ARB: angiotensin receptor blocker, CCB: calcium channel blocker, GERD: gastroesophageal reflux disease, NDRI: norepinephrine dopamine reuptake inhibitor, NSAID: non-steroidal anti-inflammatory drug, PPI: proton pump inhibitor, SNRI: serotonin norepinephrine reuptake inhibitor, SSRI: selective serotonin reuptake inhibitor.

Common Classes of Drugs for Different Diseases

The following section will discuss different classes of medications referenced in the prior tables. It is important to recognize that drugs with a similar therapeutic effect might have different mechanisms/modes of action. For example, ACE inhibitors (e.g. ramipril), calcium channel blockers (e.g. amlodipine), and antihypertensive agents have similar therapeutic effects but their mechanisms of action are different. When filling a prescription, it is important to understand how a drug works. Not only does knowledge about the pharmacology of a medicine help to identify possible drug interactions, but it also helps to facilitate patients' understanding of why medications are prescribed for them.

<u>Medications Acting on the Nervous System</u>
Antidepressants and Anxiolytics
Antidepressants are used to treat different mood disorders including depression, anxiety, phobias, and obsessive-compulsive disorder (OCD). Treatment for depression includes various medications, in addition to cognitive behavioral therapy (e.g. counseling).

The following are some of the symptoms frequently observed with depression:

- Difficulty concentrating
- Decreased interest or no interest in activities that used to be enjoyable
- Fatigue or lack of energy
- Sense of worthlessness or hopelessness
- Difficulty sleeping
- Changes in appetite
- Suicidal thoughts

Antidepressants exert their therapeutic effects by modulating the release or action of various neurotransmitters in the brain. Neurotransmitters are chemical messengers that transmit signals from one neuron to another. The common side effects of antidepressants are serotonin syndrome (headache, agitation, tremor, hallucination, tachycardia, hyperthermia, shivering and sweating), sexual dysfunction, weight changes, gastric acidity, diarrhea, sleep disturbances, and suicidal ideation.

Commonly prescribed antidepressant medications include:

- Sertraline
- Fluoxetine
- Paroxetine
- Citalopram
- Escitalopram
- Venlafaxine
- Desvenlafaxine
- Duloxetine
- Trazadone
- Bupropion
- Amitriptyline
- Nortriptyline

Benzodiazepines are a class of medications used for the short-term treatment of anxiety. They are often combined with antidepressants during initial treatment to increase treatment compliance. Benzodiazepines have the potential for significant physical dependence and withdrawal symptoms. These drugs can be used as sedatives and hypnotics and are also utilized as an add-on therapy with anti-convulsant medications. Benzodiazepines are often used to treat symptoms from alcohol withdrawal. The majority of benzodiazepines are labeled as Class IV controlled substances. The common side effects of these medications include physical dependence, sedation, drowsiness, dizziness, and lack of coordination.

The following are commonly prescribed benzodiazepines:

- Diazepam
- Lorazepam
- Clonazepam
- Alprazolam
- Midazolam
- Temazepam

Antipsychotics
Antipsychotics are used to treat psychosis, including schizophrenia and bipolar disorder. Psychosis is often characterized by a cluster of symptoms including delusions (false beliefs), paranoia (fear or anxiety), hallucinations, and disordered thoughts. The most common side effects of antipsychotics are dyskinesia (movement disorder), loss of libido or sex drive, gynecomastia (breast enlargement) in males, weight gain, heart diseases (QT prolongation), and metabolic disorders including type 2 diabetes.

The following are examples of commonly prescribed antipsychotics:

- Chlorpromazine
- Fluphenazine
- Haloperidol
- Aripiprazole
- Olanzapine
- Risperidone

- Ziprasidone
- Clozapine

Stimulant Medications
Stimulant medications are also called sympathomimetic agents, as they work by augmenting the sympathetic neurotransmitter activity (e.g. epinephrine and norepinephrine). These drugs are often used during emergencies to treat cardiac arrest and shock. Stimulant medications are more commonly used to treat attention-deficit hyperactivity disorder (ADHD). The common side effects of such medications include irritability, weight loss, insomnia, dizziness, agitation, headache, abdominal pain, tachycardia, growth retardation, hypertension, and cardiovascular disturbances, and death.

The following are examples of sympathomimetic drugs that are used in the treatment of ADHD:

- Methylphenidate
- Dextroamphetamine
- Lisdexamfetamine
- Mixed salts of amphetamine
- Atomoxetine

Anticonvulsant Medications
Anticonvulsants are also called antiepileptic or anti-seizure medications. They are used in the treatment of epileptic seizure. They suppress excessive firing of neurons and therefore, prevent the initiation and spread of seizures. This class of medications is often used to stabilize mood in bipolar disorder or for the treatment of neuropathic pain. The common side effects are dizziness, sedation, weight gain, hepatotoxicity, hair loss, blood disorders, etc. Anticonvulsants are teratogenic and can cause significant harm to a fetus and result in birth defects. Therefore, female patients on anticonvulsant therapy should consult with their physicians before planning pregnancy.

The common medications in this class include the following:

- Carbamazepine
- Oxcarbazepine
- Phenytoin
- Valproic acid
- Divalproex
- Levetiracetam
- Lamotrigine
- Topiramate
- Clobazam

Medications Acting on the Cardiovascular System
Lipid-Lowering Medications
Lipid-lowering medications are used for the treatment of high blood lipids (hyperlipidemia), including high cholesterol (hypercholesterolemia) and high triglycerides (hypertriglyceridemia). Although a patient with hypercholesterolemia typically will not experience symptoms, the condition leads to the accumulation of fatty deposits in the blood vessels and liver, called atherosclerotic plaques. As time progresses, the deposits slow, impede, or block the flow of blood through the vessels. When blood flow is compromised to the heart muscle, ischemic heart disease can result. If the blood flow to the brain decreases, there is a possibility of ischemic stroke. Compromised blood supply in peripheral tissues and

limbs can cause the development of peripheral vascular diseases (PVD). Lifestyle changes, such as a healthy diet and regular exercise, can significantly reduce the risk of hypercholesterolemia, even in the presence of predisposing genetic risk factors. Total cholesterol is determined from two components: high-density lipoproteins (HDL) cholesterol, considered the "good" cholesterol, and low-density lipoproteins (LDL) cholesterol, considered the "bad" cholesterol. Although it is helpful to keep a lower total cholesterol level for health and reduced disease risk, it is more critical to keep the ratio of HDL to LDL elevated.

Examples of lipid-lowering agents include:

- Statins: pravastatin, simvastatin, atorvastatin, rosuvastatin
- Cholesterol absorptions inhibitors: ezetimibe, cholestyramine, colestipol
- Fibrates: Gemfibrozil, fenofibrate

Antihypertensive Medications
Antihypertensive medications are used to treat high blood pressure. Although hypertensive individuals generally do not have symptoms, some people experience headaches, blurred vision, and dizziness. When high blood pressure is left untreated, it can lead to different clinical conditions including coronary artery disease, heart failure, kidney failure, or stroke. There are two values that comprise a blood pressure measure. The top number is the systolic pressure (the pressure on the arterial walls when the heart muscle contracts) and the bottom number is the diastolic pressure (the pressure on the arterial walls when the heart muscle relaxes). Normal, healthy blood pressure in adults should be a systolic reading less than 120 mmHg and a diastolic pressure less than 80 mmHg.

There are three stages of high blood pressure, as outlined below:

- Prehypertension is characterized by systolic pressure between 120-139 mmHg and diastolic pressure between 80-89 mmHg

- Stage 1 hypertension is characterized by systolic pressure between 140-159 mmHg and diastolic pressure between 90-99 mmHg

- Stage 2 hypertension is characterized by systolic pressure of 160 mmHg and higher and diastolic pressure of 100 mmHg and higher

ACE Inhibitors (ACEIs): "ACE inhibitors," or angiotensin-converting enzyme inhibitors, are used to treat hypertension and cardiovascular diseases. The most common side effect of ACE inhibitors is a chronic dry cough, which, in many cases, is so annoying for a patient that it results in switching the medication to a different class. Other frequent side effects are low blood pressure (hypotension), dizziness, fatigue, headache, and hyperkalemia (increased blood potassium levels).

Examples of some ACE Inhibitors include:

- Ramipril
- Enalapril
- Lisinopril
- Captopril
- Quinapril
- Perindopril

Angiotensin Receptor Blockers (ARBs): ARBs have similar therapeutic effects as ACE Inhibitors; however, they tend to have better compliance, due to their lower incidence of persistent cough. They block the effect of angiotensin at the receptor site and are widely used for hypertension and cardiovascular disease. The common side effects are hypotension, fatigue, dizziness, headache, and hyperkalemia.

Examples of ARBs include:

- Losartan
- Irbesartan
- Valsartan
- Candesartan
- Telmisartan
- Olmesartan

Calcium Channel Blockers (CCBs): CCBs work by decreasing calcium entry through calcium channels. By regulating the movement of calcium, contraction of vascular smooth muscle is controlled, which causes blood vessels to dilate. This reduces blood pressure and workload on the heart, so this type of medication is used to treat hypertension and angina, and to control heart rate. Common side effects of CCBs include dizziness, flushing of the face, headache, edema (swelling), tachycardia (fast heart rate), bradycardia (slow heart rate), and constipation. In combination with other medications that treat hypertension, calcium channel blocker toxicity is possible. Combinations, like verapamil with beta-blockers, can lead to severe bradycardia.

The following are examples of common calcium channel blockers:

- Amlodipine
- Nifedipine
- Felodipine
- Verapamil
- Diltiazem

Beta Blockers: Beta blockers are an important class of antihypertensive medications, and are widely used to treat hypertension and cardiovascular disease. Some of them are also used to treat migraines, agitation, and anxiety. The side effects of beta blockers include hypotension, dizziness, bradycardia, headache, bronchoconstriction (trouble breathing), and fatigue.

Commonly prescribed beta blockers include:

- Atenolol
- Metoprolol
- Propranolol
- Sotalol
- Nadolol
- Carvedilol
- Labetalol

Vasodilators: Vasodilators cause blood vessels to dilate, lowering resistance to flow and reducing the workload on the heart. Vasodilators are used to treat hypertension, angina, and heart failure. The common side effects associated with their use include lightheadedness, dizziness, low blood pressure, flushing, reflex tachycardia, and headache. Vasodilators should not be combined with medications for erectile dysfunction, as this interaction can cause a fatal drop in blood pressure.

Examples of common vasodilators include:

- Nitroglycerin (available as sublingual tablets, sprays, patches, and extended release capsules
- Isosorbide mononitrate
- Isosorbide dinitrate
- Hydralazine
- Minoxidil (limited use)

Alpha-1 Receptor Blockers: Alpha-blockers decrease the norepinephrine-induced vascular contraction, causing relaxation of blood vessels and a resultant reduction in blood pressure. This type of medication is used to treat high blood pressure and benign prostatic hyperplasia (BPH). The common side effects of this class of medications include hypotension, dizziness, headache, tachycardia, weakness, and nausea.

Examples of alpha blockers include:

- Prazosin
- Doxazosin
- Terazosin
- Tamsulosin (primarily used to treat BPH)
- Alfuzosin (primarily used to treat BPH)

Diuretics: Diuretics are used alone and in combination with other medications to treat hypertension. They are often used to eliminate excess body fluid to treat swelling/edema. Diuretics inhibit the absorption of sodium in renal tubules, resulting in increased elimination of salt and water. This action increases urine output, decreases blood volume, and lowers blood pressure. Side effects of diuretics include hypotension, dizziness, hypokalemia, dehydration, hyperglycemia, polyuria (frequent or excessive urination), fatigue, syncope (fainting), and tinnitus (ringing in ears).

Examples of commonly prescribed diuretics include:

- Furosemid
- Bumetanide
- Hydrochlorthiazide
- Spironolactone
- Amiloride
- Triamterene

Medications Acting on the Respiratory System
Antiasthmatics
Antiasthmatics are used to prevent and treat the acute symptoms of asthma, which is a disease characterized by wheezing, cough, chest tightness, and shortness of breath. Acute asthma can be life-threatening and needs to be treated promptly. Asthma is caused by inflammation and constriction of the airways, which results in difficulty breathing. Acute asthma may be exacerbated by certain triggering factors including environmental allergens, certain medications (e.g. aspirin), stress or exercise, smoke, and lung infections. It is important to avoid the triggering factors to prevent acute symptoms. The

common side effects of antiasthmatics are cough, hoarseness, decreased bone mineral density, growth retardation in children, mouth thrush, agitation, tachycardia, and a transient increase in blood pressure.

There are two categories to asthma medications that can be used alone or in combination:

1. 1. Bronchodilators (dilate the airway to ease breathing)

- Salbutamol
- Formoterol (generally used in combination with inhaled corticosteroids)
- Salmeterol (generally used in combination with inhaled corticosteroids)

2. 2. Anti-inflammatory agents

- Fluticasone (inhaled corticosteroid)
- Budesonide (inhaled corticosteroid)
- Beclometasone (inhaled corticosteroid)
- Montelukast
- Zafirlukast

Medication to Treat COPD (Chronic Obstructive Pulmonary Disease)
COPD is an obstructive airway disease that is characterized by coughing, wheezing, shortness of breath, and sputum production. COPD is a progressive disease and it worsens over time. COPD is a combination of two common conditions: chronic bronchitis and emphysema. Chronic bronchitis is inflammation of the smooth lining of bronchial tubes. These tubes are responsible for carrying air to the alveoli, which are the air sacs in the lungs responsible for gaseous exchange between the lungs and blood. Emphysema results from alveolar damage, reducing the ability for healthy gas exchange. These two pathologies cause breathing difficulties in patients with COPD. The contributing factors for the development of COPD include smoking, environmental pollutions, and genetic risk factors. The side effects of COPD medications are similar to that of antiasthmatics.

The medications commonly used to treat COPD include the following:

3. 1. Bronchodilators (dilate the airway to ease breathing)

- Salbutamol
- Formoterol (generally used in combination with inhaled corticosteroids)
- Salmeterol (generally used in combination with inhaled corticosteroids)

4. 2. Anti-inflammatory agents

- Ipratropium (Atrovent)
- Tiotropium (Spiriva)
- Fluticasone
- Budesonide

Medications Acting on the Digestive System
Gastric acid Neutralizers/Suppressants
Gastric acid neutralizers/suppressants either neutralize stomach acid or decrease acid production, and therefore, provide relief of symptoms associated with hyperacidity. They are also used to treat gastroesophageal reflux disease, or GERD. In GERD, the lower esophageal sphincter does not close

properly, which causes the contents of the stomach to back up into the esophagus. This leads to irritation, which is why the common symptoms of GERD include heartburn, coughing, nausea, difficulty swallowing, and a strained voice. There are many factors that can cause or exacerbate GERD including obesity, pregnancy, eating a large meal, acidic foods, a hiatal hernia, and smoking. Lifestyle modifications such as avoiding trigger foods, losing weight (if obesity is a component), decreasing meal size, and trying not to lie down immediately after eating, can reduce symptoms.

The medications used to treat hyperacidity in stomach include the following:

- Antacids (e.g. calcium carbonate)
- Ranitidine
- Famotidine
- Omeprazole
- Esomeprazole
- Lansoprazole
- Rabeprazole
- Pantoprazole

Medications Acting on the Endocrine System
Anti-Diabetic Medications
Anti-diabetic medications are used to treat diabetes, which is a chronic metabolic disease in which the body cannot properly regulate blood sugar levels. This dysregulation is caused by either inadequate or absent insulin production from the pancreas (Type 1 diabetes) or inadequate action of insulin in peripheral tissues (i.e. insulin resistance in Type 2 diabetes). Type 1 diabetes usually occurs in early childhood and is typically treated with insulin injections or medications. Type 2 diabetes generally develops later in adolescence or adulthood, and is related to poor diet, lack of physical activity, and obesity. Diabetes often does not to cause daily symptoms, but symptoms do arise when blood sugar is either too high (from inadequate control) or too low (from inappropriate dosing of hypoglycemic (antidiabetic) agents, including insulin). A few of the symptoms of diabetes include increased thirst and hunger, fatigue, blurred vision, a tingling sensation in the feet, and frequent urination.

Examples of some antidiabetic medications include:

- Insulin
- Metformin
- Acarbose
- Gliclazide, glyburide, glimepiride
- Rosiglitazone, pioglitazone
- Sitagliptin, saxagliptin

Drug and Non-Drug Therapy in Type 2 Diabetes: The most effective way of treating Type 2 diabetes is to combine both drug and non-drug therapies. As a part of the treatment, drug therapy can stimulate the pancreas to produce more insulin or help the body better use the insulin produced by the pancreas. As part of the non-drug therapy, counseling is necessary to help patients understand the important diet and lifestyle modifications. Patients with Type 2 diabetes should try to decrease their consumption of processed foods, simple carbohydrates and refined sugars, and overall caloric intake, while increasing physical activity. These interventions help to decrease the requirement of antidiabetic medications and prevent long-term diabetes-related complications.

Glucometer: Patients with diabetes should test their blood sugar regularly to ensure that it is well-controlled. Glucometers are used to measure blood sugar. Patients insert a testing strip into the glucometer, prick a finger with a lancet, and then apply a drop of blood to the test strip. Upon applying the blood, the meter gives a blood sugar reading. Most modern machines need a very small amount of blood to obtain an accurate reading and can generate the result in seconds. Some more advanced meters can store readings for a period of time, so patients can present it to their physicians for review.

Female Hormones
Hormonal medications are generally used as oral contraceptives to prevent pregnancy. Female hormonal medications are also used to treat premenstrual symptoms (PMS), post-menopausal symptoms, acne, and endometriosis. They are also used as emergency contraceptives to prevent unwanted and accidental pregnancy. Oral contraceptives can provide hormones (estrogen and/or progestin), which suppress the egg maturation and ovulation process. Additionally, hormonal contraceptives prevent the endometrium from thickening in preparation to hold the fertilized egg. A mucus barrier is created by progestin, which stops the sperm from migrating to the fallopian tubes and fertilizing the egg.

There are many side effects associated with oral contraceptives, including increasing the risk of fatal blood clots, especially in women older than 35 or in women who smoke. More common and less severe side effects include:

- Nausea and stomach upset
- Headache
- Weight gain
- Spotting between periods
- Mood changes
- Lighter periods
- Aching or swollen breasts

More serious side effects that need immediate emergency care include:

- Chest pain
- Blurred vision
- Stomach pain
- Severe headaches

Examples of some commercially available brands of contraceptive include:

- Yasmin
- Ortho Tri-Cyclin
- TriNessa
- Sprintec
- Ovcon
- Plan B (emergency contraceptive)

<u>Medications Acting on the Immune System</u>
Antivirals
Antivirals are used to fight viruses in the body, by either stopping replication or blocking the function of a viral protein. They are used to treat HIV, herpes, hepatitis B and C, and influenza, among other viruses.

Vaccines are also available to prevent some viral infections. Side effects of antivirals include headache, nausea, blood abnormalities including anemia and neutropenia (low neutrophil count), dizziness, cough, runny or stuff nose, etc.

Some examples of disease-specific antivirals include:

- Acyclovir, valaciclovir (Valtrex): Herpes simplex, herpes zoster, and herpes B
- Ritonavir, indinavir, darunavir: Protease inhibitor for HIV
- Tenofovir (Viread): Hepatitis B and HIV infection
- Interferon: Hepatitis C
- Oseltamivir (Tamiflu): Influenza

Antibiotics
Antibiotics are antimicrobial agents that are used for treatment and prevention of bacterial infections. The mechanism of action of an antibiotic involves either killing bacteria or inhibiting their growth. Antibiotics are not effective against viruses, and therefore, they should not be used to treat viral infections. Antibiotics are often prescribed based on the result of a bacterial culture to ascertain which class of antibiotic(s) the respective strain will respond to. The common side effects of antibiotics include allergies, hypersensitivity reactions or anaphylaxis, stomach upset, diarrhea, candida (fungal) infections, and bacterial resistance (superinfection, in which a strain of bacteria develops resistance to a broad classes of antibiotics).

Commonly prescribed antibiotics include:

- Penicillin V
- Amoxicillin (with or without clavulinic acid)
- Ampicillin
- Cloxacillin
- Cephalexin
- Cefuroxime
- Cefixime
- Tetracyclin
- Doxycyline
- Minocycline
- Gentamycin
- Tobramycin
- Ciprofloxacin
- Levofloxacin
- Erythromycin
- Azithromycin
- Clarithromycin
- Clindamycin

Antimetabolites
Antimetabolites are used to treat diseases including severe psoriasis, rheumatoid arthritis, and several types of cancer (breast, lung, lymphoma, and leukemia). The most commonly used medication of this class is methotrexate, which suppresses the growth of abnormal cells and the action of the immune system. Methotrexate is widely used to treat rheumatoid arthritis. This medication is typically

prescribed as once a week dose, and it should not be prescribed for daily dosing because overdosing can be lethal. Pharmacists should be alerted to any prescriptions for daily methotrexate, as the doctor must be contacted to confirm and correct the dosing.

The following are the potential side effects of methotrexate:

- Dizziness
- Drowsiness
- Headache
- Swollen gums
- Increased susceptibility to infections
- Hair loss
- Confusion
- Weakness

Steroids

Steroids are used to treat allergies, asthma, rashes, swelling, and inflammation. These medications are available in different forms, such as oral tablets, nasal sprays, eye drops, topical creams and ointments, inhalants, and injections. The common side effects of steroids include insulin resistance and diabetes, osteoporosis, depression, hypertension, edema, glaucoma, etc.

The following are examples of commonly prescribed corticosteroids:

- Prednisone
- Hydrocortisone
- Fluticason
- Triamcinolone
- Mometasone
- Budesonide
- Fluocinolone
- Betamethasone
- Dexamethasone

Total Parenteral Nutrition: Total parenteral nutrition is used in situations where a patient cannot orally ingest food or digest food through the stomach and intestines. In such cases, total parental nutrition is essential to maintain patient nourishment and to prevent wasting or malnutrition.

The clinical conditions requiring total parenteral nutrition include the following:

- Any cause of malnourishment
- Failure of liver or kidneys
- Short bowel syndrome
- Severe burns
- Enterocutaneous fistulas
- Sepsis
- Chemotherapy and radiation
- Neonates
- Conditions requiring full bowel rest, such as pancreatitis, ulcerative colitis, or Crohn's disease

Therapeutic Equivalence

There are certain parameters (bioavailability, dosage form, active ingredients, safety profile, and clinical efficacy) that need to be identical or nearly identical to ensure that a specific medication and the reference medication are equivalent. The extent that one medication can be substituted for another depends on which type of equivalence (bio, pharmaceutical, and therapeutic) has been established. Therefore, pharmacy technicians must understand the different types of equivalence.

Pharmaceutical Equivalents
Pharmaceutical equivalents refer to two or more medications that have equal quantities/strength of the identical active ingredients in the same dosage form, and with the same route of administration. The active ingredients in pharmaceutical equivalent formulations should meet the official compendia (e.g. USP and NF) standard on identity, purity, strength, and quality. Pharmaceutical equivalent formulations, however, may vary in shape, scoring configuration, packaging, excipients (preservatives, colors, and flavors), labeling, and date of expiration.

Pharmaceutical Alternatives
Pharmaceutical alternatives refer to medications that have the same therapeutic moiety (structure), but are formulated as different salts, esters, or complexes. They might have different strengths and dosage forms. For example, tetracycline 250 mg formulated as hydrochloride and phosphate salts are pharmaceutical alternatives. Generally, different dosage forms and strengths of a single medication by a single manufacturer are pharmaceutical alternatives. The extended release formulations and the standard/immediate release formulations are, therefore, pharmaceutical alternatives, as they carry the same active ingredient.

Bioequivalents
Bioequivalents refer to two or more pharmaceutically-comparable products that demonstrate equivalent bioavailability when tested under similar experimental conditions. The rate and extent of absorption of bioequivalent products should be identical. Bioequivalence of two or more formulations is determined by comparing the rate and extent of absorption of those formulations with that of the reference standard formulation.

Therapeutic Equivalents
Therapeutic equivalents refer to two or more pharmaceutical products that provide identical clinical effect, safety, and efficacy. Pharmaceutical equivalents should meet the following criteria:

1. They should have identical safety and efficacy

2. They should be pharmaceutically-equivalent

3. They should be bioequivalent

4. They should be adequately labeled

5. They should be manufactured in accordance with the standards of Current Good Manufacturing Practice (cGMP)

Bioavailability
Bioavailability is a function of the rate and extent of absorption of a drug from a formulation. It is the fraction of a drug that reaches the blood circulation after administration. The bioavailability following an intravenous administration is 100%, since the medication is completely available in circulation.

The following are parameters which measure bioavailability on a concentration-time curve:

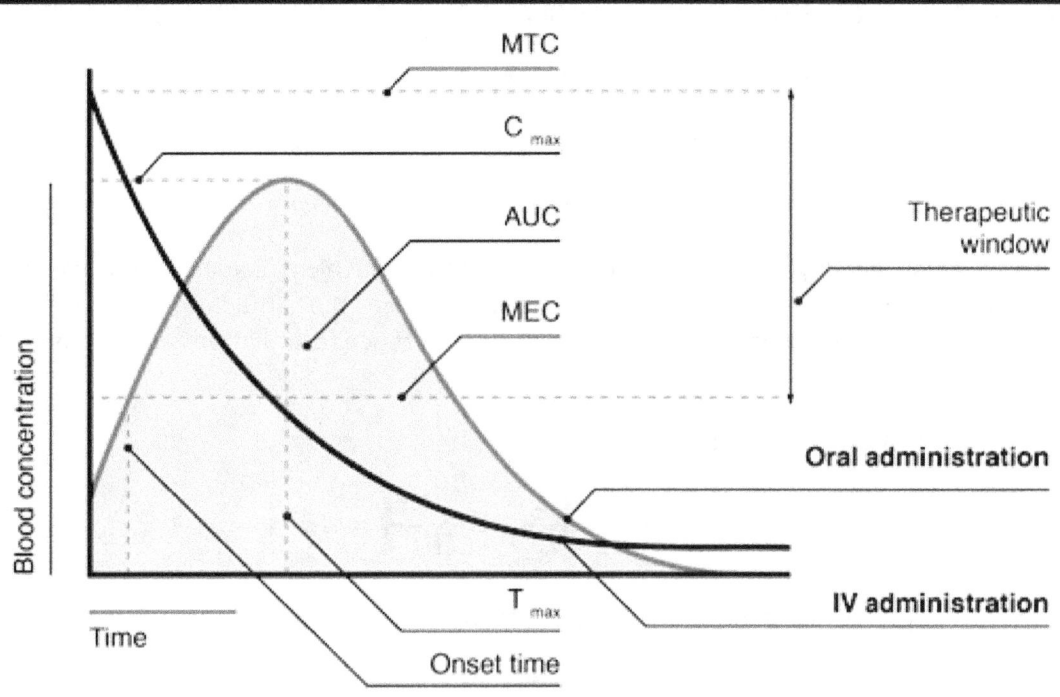

- C_{max}: The peak blood concentration of the medication.

- T_{max}: The time to reach the peak blood concentration of the medication; indicative of the rate of absorption of a drug from a formulation

- *MEC*: The minimum effective concentration, i.e. the minimum drug concentration required to exhibit the therapeutic effect

- *MTC*: The maximum therapeutic concentration at which the greatest therapeutic effect of a drug is achieved

- *Therapeutic window*: The range of drug concentrations between which the desired therapeutic effect is obtained without any significant toxicity

- *AUC*: The area under the concentration-time curve; refers to the amount of the drug absorbed in the system following administration. It is the principle index of the bioavailability of a drug from a dosage form.

Below are explanations of two types of bioavailability:

- *Absolute bioavailability*: This refers to the comparison between the bioavailability of a drug following a non-intravenous route (e.g. oral, rectal, sublingual, subcutaneous, transdermal, etc.) of administration and the bioavailability of the same drug following intravenous administration. It is measured by the ratio of AUC from the non-IV route to that of the IV route.

- So, % absolute bioavailability is:

$$F_{abs} = \frac{AUC_{PO}}{D_{PO}} \times \frac{D_{IV}}{AUC_{IV}} \times 100$$

Where, AUC_{po} = AUC from oral administration

AUC_{iv} = AUC from intravenous administration

D_{po} = dose of oral formulation

D_{iv} = dose of intravenous formulation

- *Relative bioavailability*: This refers to the comparison of the bioavailability of a drug from one dosage form (e.g. tablet or capsule) to the bioavailability of the same drug from a reference dosage form (e.g. syrup or suspension). When the reference formulation is an IV dosage form, it also indicates absolute bioavailability.

- So, % relative bioavailability is:

$$F_{rel} = \frac{AUC_A}{D_A} \times \frac{D_B}{AUC_B} \times 100$$

Where, AUC_A = AUC from formulation A (test formulation)

AUC_B = AUC from formulation B (reference standard)

D_A = dose of formulation A (test formulation)

D_B = dose of formulation B (reference standard)

Generic Substitution

Generic substitution refers to filling a prescription with a generic, therapeutically-equivalent formulation instead of an original brand name formulation. For example, the generic form of Lipitor® is Atorvastatin; both have the same clinical efficacy and safety for treating high cholesterol. Dispensing generic Atorvastatin for a prescription written for Lipitor® is an example of generic substitution. There are different laws in each state for filling prescriptions with generic substitutions, and therefore, it is important to know and abide by the laws in the state of employment.

Generally, generic medications are less expensive for patients. Prescribers may deem the brand name medically necessary and order "dispense as written" or "no substitution" to prevent generic substitutions. It is also important to check the therapeutic index of a drug before substituting with a generic medication. Drugs with a narrow therapeutic index should be cautiously dispensed as generics, as minute changes in bioavailability can impose significant toxicity. Examples of such drugs include levothyroxine, lithium, warfarin, phenytoin, and digoxin.

Therapeutic Substitutions

Therapeutic substitution can be done in two different forms: substitution of an equally potent drug from within the same class or substitution of a drug from a different class of drugs, but with the same pharmacologic effect and similar potency yet a different mechanism of action. An example of the first type of substitution is dispensing enalapril for lisinopril, which is substitution of an ACE inhibitor with another ACE inhibitor. An example of the second type of substitution is giving enalapril in place of amlodipine, which is substituting a calcium channel blocker with an ACE inhibitor, where both drugs have similar antihypertensive effect but different modes of action. The frequency of therapeutic substitutions is low in community pharmacies and is more likely to happen in hospitals or federal facilities. It is imperative to make sure that these types of substitutions are discussed with the prescriber before making the substitution.

There are several consequences of therapeutic substitutions:

- Either over- or under-treating the patient
- The unfavorable effects either get better or worse
- There could be different adverse effects
- The cost of the prescription could be higher or lower for the patient

Orange Book
Orange Book is a reference to find drugs that have been approved and evaluated for therapeutic equivalence. The official name of the book is *Approved Drug Products with Therapeutic Equivalence Evaluations*, and it is now available online at the FDA's website.

Drug Interactions

Drug interaction refers to the alteration in pharmacology (absorption, distribution, metabolism, elimination, efficacy, side effects, etc.) of a medication by various factors including disease conditions, prescription and OTC medications, and foods or nutritional supplements. These interactions may result in either an augmentation or decrease in the efficacy and/or toxicity of the respective medication. Drug interaction should be carefully reviewed in order to avoid serious life-threatening conditions.

Examples of different types of drug interactions and examples within each type are described below.

Drug-Disease Interactions
NSAIDS and Peptic Ulcers
NSAIDs including aspirin, ibuprofen, naproxen, and indomethacin can cause stomach irritation and can aggravate peptic ulcer symptoms. Therefore, NSAIDs should not be used by patients with peptic ulcers or GERD. If NSAIDs are used by patients with hyperacidity, gastro-protective agents, such as proton pumps inhibitors (e.g. omeprazole, pantoprazole, lansoprazole, etc.), should also be used.

Diuretics and Diabetes
Diuretics are used to treat hypertension and edema. Hydrochlorthiazide is a commonly prescribed diuretic that can cause glucose intolerance and hyperglycemia. Therefore, if a patient with type 2 diabetes is prescribed a diuretic, blood sugar control becomes difficult, so routine monitoring of blood sugar is required. If blood sugar is not properly controlled, dose adjustments of the anti-diabetic medication or alternative diuretics should be considered.

Drug-Drug Interactions
Warfarin and NSAIDs
Warfarin is a commonly prescribed blood thinner, indicated to prevent blood clots in various cardiovascular diseases. Patients on warfarin should not take other prescription/OTC/herbal medications without consulting with their prescriber and pharmacist. For example, commonly available OTC NSAIDs can cause an increase in the blood-thinning effect of warfarin and result in internal hemorrhage.

The following medications can interact with warfarin:

- Aspirin
- Acetaminophen (at high doses)
- Ibuprofen
- Naproxen
- Celecoxib
- Diclofenac
- Indomethacin
- Piroxicam

Oral Contraceptives and Antibiotics
Antibiotics can decrease the effect hormonal oral contraceptives and cause accidental pregnancy. Non-hormonal back-up methods, such as condoms, should be used while a woman taking an oral contraceptive is prescribed an antibiotic. Other medications that can affect the efficacy of oral contraceptives include anti-fungals, a few anti-seizure medications, certain HIV medications, and a few herbal preparations, like St. John's Wort.

Nitroglycerin and Erectile Dysfunction Medications
Nitroglycerin is a vasodilator that is often used to treat episodes of angina. To prevent recurring angina, the extended release capsules of nitroglycerin are taken daily, whereas in cases of non-frequent occurrence, sublingual tablets or sprays can be used. Medications to treat erectile dysfunctions, such as sildenafil, tadalafil, and vardenafil, should not be taken with nitroglycerin. These medications augment the vasodilatory effect of nitroglycerin and can lead to irreversible hypotension and fatality. Emergency care should be sought immediately if this combination accidentally happens. The symptoms of hypotension include dizziness, fainting, and cold, clammy skin.

Drug-Food and Drug-Nutrient Interactions
Statins and Grapefruit Juice
Statins (e.g. pravastatin, simvastatin, atorvastatin, and rosuvastatin) are used to treat hypocholesteremia. Patients taking this medication should avoid drinking grapefruit juice or consuming large amounts of grapefruit because this juice decreases the metabolism of statins, resulting in a buildup of statins in the body. The risk of serious side effects is increased when statin buildup occurs, with possible resultant muscle or liver damage. Pharmacists should counsel patients about avoiding grapefruit juice while on statins. Although increasing statin dosage may seem to benefit the patient, the liver can only process so much. Accumulation of a statin in the body can cause muscle damage, pain, and rhabdomyolysis—a serious and potentially lethal side effect. In rhabdomyolysis, the skeletal muscle is rapidly catabolized. Patients taking statins should undergo routine blood tests and notify their doctors immediately about symptoms of muscle pain or fatigue. Undetected and unmanaged rhabdomyolysis can result in death.

MAOIs and Tyramine
Monoamine oxidase inhibitors (MAOIs) are used to treat chronic depression that does not respond to other medications or treatments. Due to side effects and drug interactions, MAOIs are not commonly prescribed. Examples of MAOIs are phenelzine (Nardil®), selegiline (Emsam®), and tranylcypromine (Parnate®). MAOIs can cause serotonin syndrome. There are many medications and foods that can lead to severe side effects when combined with MAOIs. Foods like wine, cheese, certain meats, and pickled foods carry tyramine, which leads to spikes in blood pressure, if co-administered with MAOIs.

Drug-OTC Interactions
Antihypertensives and Decongestants
Pseudoephedrine and phenylephrine are used as decongestants in different OTC cough and cold medications. These medications have sympathomimetic effects and can cause elevated blood pressure. Therefore, if a decongestant medication is taken by patients on antihypertensive medication, it reduces the blood pressure control of the antihypertensive agent. Hypertensive patients should avoid taking OTC medications containing sympathomimetic agents.

Antihistamines and Sedatives
OTC antihistamines, such as diphenhydramine and chlorpheniramine, are used to treat various allergic conditions. Antihistamines can cause sedation and drowsiness, which can potentiate the side effects of sedatives and hypnotics. Patients taking sedatives—such as diazepam, lorazepam, alprazolam, and midazolam—should be cautious when taking an OTC antihistamine.

Drug-Laboratory Interactions
Antibiotics and Bacterial Cultures
Treatment with certain medications can affect laboratory results. For example, the blood or urine sample collected from a patient taking an antibiotic for one infection might yield a false antibiotic sensitivity or culture report for a second infection. The lab work should, therefore, be scheduled after the wash-out period of the first antibiotic.

Polypharmacy
Polypharmacy occurs when a patient takes multiple medications to treat different medical conditions. This happens mostly in elderly patients who are being treated for several medical conditions. Polypharmacy can cause serious drug interactions. Polypharmacy also tends to happen when a patient sees multiple doctors to treat separate conditions. Pharmacy technicians can help to prevent adverse consequences of polypharmacy by alerting pharmacists to drug interactions.

Strength/Dose, Dosage Forms, Physical Appearance, Routes of Administration, and Duration of Drug Therapy

Dose, Dosage Forms, and Physical Appearance
The list below shows the different dosage abbreviations and their meanings:

- cap = capsule
- tab = tablet
- gtt = drop
- i, ii, iii, iv = 1, 2, 3, 4 (quantities are often identified with roman numerals on prescriptions)
- mg = milligrams
- mL = milliliter
- tbsp. = tablespoon (15 mL)
- tsp. = teaspoon (5 mL)
- ss = one-half
- mcg/ ug = microgram

Note that *ug* is not being used as much anymore, as it is confused with *mg*. If unsure, pharmacy technicians should check with the prescriber.

A pharmaceutical dosage form is a formulation type in which the active ingredient(s) (with excipients) is manufactured to be administered to patients. There are different types of pharmaceuticals dosage forms, some of which include the following:

1. Tablets are the most common oral dosage form. Tablets can be made from firmly condensed powder into the desired shape. Tablets are often coated to mask a bad taste/smell of a medication. There are also more complex types of tablets that are designed by using special polymers, which release the medication from the tablet core in a controlled pattern, often in slow-release formulations.

2. Capsules can use a hard or soft shell, which contains powder or liquid ingredients inside. Most capsules are made from gelatin, a collagen by-product of an animal protein. Other capsule shells contain plant-based polysaccharides such as carrageenan, modified starch, and cellulose.

3. Liquid formulations are primarily of two categories: elixirs and suspensions. An elixir is a clear liquid solution in which active ingredients are mixed in a liquid carrier (or formulation vehicle); shaking is *not* required to mix the ingredients. In suspensions, medication is suspended in a liquid carrier. It is essential to shake suspensions before administration, as some ingredients often collect at the bottom as sediment. Sometimes a suspension is supplied as a dry power, which needs to be mixed with the appropriate volume of distilled water, before dispensing it to the patient.

4. Suppositories are solid dosage forms that are inserted into body cavities, including the rectum, vagina, and urethra, where they melt and provide local or systemic effects. Due to local administration, suppositories show fewer side effects compared to orally-administered medications. Suppositories also provide greater absorption of the medication, as they bypass the first pass metabolism in the liver.

5. An injectable is a pharmaceutical dosage form that follows the parenteral route to administer a medication locally or systemically. An injectable is manufactured in an aseptic environment and must be sterile in nature. Examples of some types of injectable routes are intravenous, intradermal, subcutaneous, intramuscular, intraperitoneal, intrathecal, intracardiac, epidural, etc.

Pharmacokinetics

Pharmacokinetics is the study of the fate of a medication in the body. The knowledge of a medication's pharmacokinetics helps to determine dosing. Pharmacokinetics of a medication includes four parameters: absorption, distribution, metabolism, and elimination. Absorption refers to the process of the medication entering blood circulation. Distribution is the process of dispersion of the medication throughout the body, including the site of action. Metabolism is the process of degradation of the parent molecule into different metabolites. Elimination refers to the process of removal of the parent molecule and the metabolites from the body.

The pharmacokinetic of a medication can be affected by various factors including:

- Age
- Race
- Gender
- Genetic factors
- Dosage form
- Disease conditions

- Foods
- Concurrent administration of other conditions

Pharmacodynamics

Pharmacodynamics refers to the study of the effects of a medication at the site of action. This helps to ascertain the mechanism of action of a medication and to determine the dose-response relationship by analyzing the interaction of a drug with its receptors at the target organ or site.

Half-Life

Half-life is a pharmacokinetic parameter that represents the unit of time over which the concentration of a medication in circulation drops to half of its initial concentration. For example, if a medication has a half-life of 15 hours, blood concentration of the drug decreases 50% every 15 hours. The longer a medication's half-life, the longer the effects persist; therefore, lower therapeutic doses or longer dosing intervals should be used. Medications in the same therapeutic class might have different half-lives, resulting in varying durations of action. Knowledge of a medication's half-life helps to determine the necessary dosage and the frequency of administration.

A medication's half-life depends on the elimination rate kinetics of the respective medication. There are two common types of elimination rate kinetics that are studied in pharmacology: first order kinetics and zero order kinetics.

First Order Kinetics
When a medication follows first order elimination kinetics, the medication undergoes a linear rate of elimination in proportion to its concentration. However, the elimination half-life remains constant independent of the initial concentration of the reactant. The metabolism and elimination of most of the drugs follow first order kinetics. Below is an example in which an IV administration of a medication follows first order kinetics with a constant half-life (i.e. $t_1 = t_2 = t_3$).

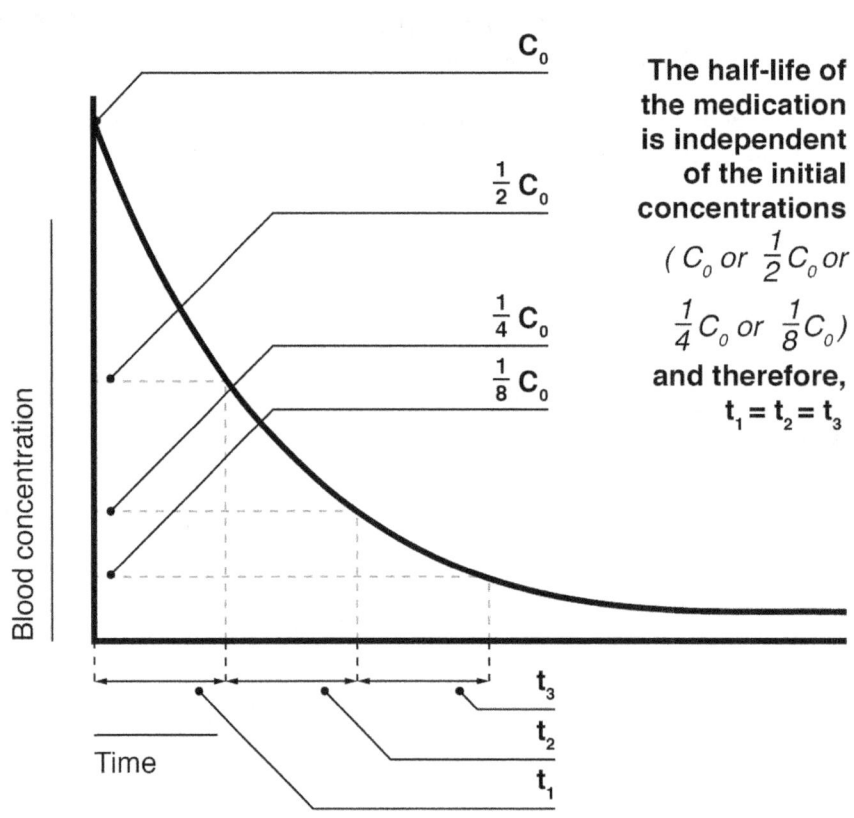

Zero Order Kinetics
Zero order kinetics refers to a reaction that proceeds at a rate independent of the concentrations of the reactants. For example, alcohol metabolism in the liver follows zero order kinetics.

Routes of Administration and Duration of Therapy
There are different routes of administration for medications including the following:

- Orally or by mouth: oral tablets, capsules, liquid preparations (elixirs and suspensions)
- Nasally: sprays or drips
- Intravenously (IV): goes through the veins and must be liquid

- Intramuscularly (IM: goes into the muscle and must be liquid
- Subcutaneously: usually an injection under the skin
- Epidurally: may be infused into epidural space in the spinal cord
- Transdermal route: medication is absorbed through the skin via patches and creams
- Rectally: these usually are suppositories and some cream medications
- Sublingually: under the tongue
- Inhalation route: many sprays and nebulizer solutions are inhaled into the lungs
- Ocular route: into the eye, usually in the form of solutions and suspensions
- Aurally: into the ear, usually in the form of solutions and suspensions

Common abbreviations for administration of medications include:

- *au* = both ears
- *as* = left ear
- *ad* = right ear
- *ou* = both eyes
- *od* = right eye
- *os* = left eye
- *po* = by mouth
- *c* = with
- *sl* = sublingual (under tongue)
- *top* = topically (apply to skin)

The following are common abbreviations found in medication directions:

- *od* = once a day
- *bid* = twice a day
- *tid* = three times a day
- *prn* = as needed
- *qd* = everyday/ daily
- *q4h/q4°* = every 4 hours
- *qid* = four times a day
- *qod* = every day
- *eod* = every other day
- *ac* = before eating (meals)
- *hs* = at bedtime
- *pc* = after eating (meals)

<u>Converting Liquid Measurements</u>
Converting Between Teaspoons, Tablespoons, and mL
It is important for patients to measure the dose when prescribed liquid medications that require a spoon or an oral syringe. One teaspoon is equal to 5 mL, and one tablespoon is equal to 15 mL.

Some examples of equivalent liquid measurements are shown below:

- 1.5 tsp. = 7.5 mL
- 2 tbsp. = 30 mL
- 10 mL = 2 tsp.

- 0.5 tbsp. = 7.5 mL
- 2.5 mL = 0.5 tsp

Converting Between mL and Ounces
It is important to use a graduated cylinder when measuring a liquid drug, and to pour with caution to measure the exact amount. A liquid ounce is equal to 30 mL. Below are some examples of equivalent measurements:

- 270 mL = 9 ounces
- 3 ounces = 90 mL
- 12 ounces = 360 mL
- 240 mL = 8 ounces

Converting Between Cups, Pints, Quarts, and Gallons
The following allow for conversions between the above-mentioned measurements:

- 2 cups = 1 pint
- 2 pints = 1 quart
- 4 quarts = 1 gallon
- 1 cup = 8 ounces
- 1 pint = 16 ounces
- 1 quart = 32 ounces
- 1 gallon = 128 ounces

Converting Between Grams, Pounds, and Kilograms
- 1 kilogram = 1000 grams
- 1 kilogram = 2.205 pounds
- 1 pound = 454 grams
- 2 pounds = 908 grams
- 227 grams = 0.5 pounds
- 681 grams = 1.5 pounds

Converting Between Grams and Ounces
One ounce is equal to 28.35 grams.

- 14.18 grams = 0.5 ounce
- 85 grams = 3 ounces
- 1.5 ounces = 42.5 grams
- 4 ounces = 113.4 grams

Converting Between Drops and mL
One mL has 20 drops. "gtt" stands for drops.

- 2 gtt ou bid x 10 days = 4 mL (2 drops in each eye twice daily for 10 days)
- 4 gtt sl q4h x 7 days = 8.4 mL (4 drops sublingually every 4 hours, i.e. 6 times a day, for 7 days)
- 5 gtt os qd x 15 days = 3.75 mL (5 drops in the left eye every day for 15 days)

Most medications that are dispensed in drops come in 5mL, 10 mL, or 15 mL bottles. It is standard practice to dispense the whole bottle, although it may be more than what is needed for the duration of treatment. Calculating the total quantity needed for the duration of treatment is required for insurance purposes, and to figure out how many or which size bottle is needed to cover the treatment.

Converting Between Grains and Milligrams
Each grain is equal to 65 milligrams.

- 3 grains = 195 mg
- 1.5 grains = 97.5 mg
- 650 mg = 10 grains
- 162.5 mg = 2.5 grains

Converting Between Celsius and Fahrenheit
The following is the formula used to convert degrees Fahrenheit to Celsius:

$$°C = (°F - 32) \times \frac{5}{9}$$

The following is the formula used to convert Celsius to Fahrenheit:

$$°F = \left(°C \times \frac{9}{5}\right) + 32$$

Examples:

- 32 °F = 0 °C
- 40 °F = 4.45 °C
- 20 °C = 68 °F
- 60 °C = 140 °F

Pediatric Dosage Rules
It is important to check and compare the dosage for children relative to that of adults, as the physician may request a dose that a manufacturer does not supply.

The following formula is used to calculate pediatric doses:

5. Dose calculation related to age:

- Young's Rule: This formula depends on age to calculate the dose, and is preferably used for children between 1-12 years of age:

- $Child\ dose = Adult\ dose \times \frac{Age\ in\ years}{(Age+12)}$

    Example: A child is 12 years old and the adult dose of the medicine is 500 mg:

- $Child\ dose = 500\ mg \times \frac{12}{(12+12)} = 250\ mg$

- Drilling's Rule: This formula uses the age of the child expressed in years:

- $Child\ dose = Adult\ dose \times \frac{Age\ in\ years}{(20)}$

Example: A child is 10 years old and the adult dose of the medicine is 750 mg:

- $Child\ dose = 750\ mg \times \dfrac{10}{(20)} = 375\ mg$

- Fried's Rule: This formula is better to use in infants until 2 years of age, and the age of the child is expressed in months:

- $Child\ dose = Adult\ dose \times \dfrac{Age\ in\ months}{(150)}$

Example: A child is 8 months old and the adult dose is 250 mg:

- $Child\ dose = 250\ mg \times \dfrac{8}{(150)} = 13.33\ mg$

6. Dose calculation related to body weight:

- Clark's Rule: This is based on weight in pounds (not kg) and can be calculated with the formula below:
- $Child\ dose = Adult\ dose \times \dfrac{Body\ weight\ in\ lb}{(150)}$

Example: A child weighs 80 pounds and the adult dose is 500 mg:

- $Child\ dose = 500\ mg \times \dfrac{80}{(150)} = 266.7\ mg$

7. Dose calculation related to body surface area:

A child's dose can also be calculated relative to body surface area (BSA). This approach is distinguished by obtaining a more representative measure of metabolic mass instead of body weight, as it is not affected as much by unusual amounts of fat. Note that an average adult with a weight of 70 kg and a height 175 cm has a body surface area of approximately 1.85 m^2.

- $Child\ dose = Adult\ dose \times \dfrac{Child's\ BSA}{Average\ adult's\ BSA}$

Body surface area (BSA) can be calculated using Mosteller's equation as follows.

$$BSA\ (m^2) = \sqrt{\dfrac{(Height\ (cm) \times Weight\ (kg))}{3600}}$$

For example, a prescription comes as 600 mg/m^2 of drug "X" for a 32-month old boy. The boy weighs 30 lbs (13.6 kg) and is 30 inches (76.2 cm) tall. What dosage should the boy receive?

$$BSA\ (m^2) = \sqrt{\dfrac{(76.2\ cm \times 13.6\ kg)}{3600}} = \sqrt{.28} = 0.53\ m^2$$

Therefore, the child's dose = 600 mg × 0.53 = 318 mg

Proportional Calculations

Proportional calculations are often used in the pharmacy to determine how much of a medication should be dispensed, to calculate a dose, or to measure the amount in compounding.

Proportional calculations are usually conducted as follows:

$$\frac{A}{B} = \frac{X}{C}$$

For example, the following prescription may be received: Amoxicillin suspension, 300 mg bid x 10 days. When checking the shelf, the only concentration available is 200 mg/5 mL. To find the dose, the equation should be set up as:

$$\frac{5\ mL}{200\ mg} = \frac{X}{300\ mg}$$

$$X = \frac{5\ mL \times 300\ mg}{200\ mg} = 7.5\ mL$$

Proportion Technique

The following steps should be used to solve a dilution problem while using the proportional technique:

- Set up the proportion equation
- Solve for x, which is the total number of units of active ingredient in the solution
- Calculate the amount of diluted solution that should be made using proportions
- Calculate x to obtain the total amount of diluted solution that can be made

To find how much diluent to add, the technician needs to subtract the original amount of solution from the total amount of diluted solution.

Example: How much sterile water should be used to dilute 1L of 70% alcohol solution to 40% solution? How much of the 40% solution is made in total?

$$\frac{70\%}{1000\ mL} = \frac{40\%}{X}$$

$$X = \frac{1000\ mL \times 40\%}{70\%} = 571.4\ mL$$

In the final step, 1000 mL – 571.4 mL = 428.6 mL of sterile water is added to 571.4 mL of the 70% solution, to make a total of 1L.

V/V, W/W and W/V Concentrations

There are different ways that concentrations can be expressed, for example, as a ratio of weight, volume, or percentage. The following ratios are used to present a concentration: V/V, W/W, and W/V. The unit for a V/V ratio is mL, as this represents a volume/volume ratio. The unit for a W/W ratio is grams, as this represents a weight/weight ratio. The measurement unit for W/V is grams/mL, as this represents weight/volume ratio.

Examples are:

- V/V = 1:500 = 1 mL/500 mL = 0.2%
- W/W = 5:100 = 5 grams/100 grams = 5%
- W/V = 10/100 = 10 grams/100 mL = 10%

Alligation Method

This method is also commonly called the *Tic-Tac-Toe method*, because it uses a grid that looks similar to a tic-tac-toe grid. The problem is set up by placing the desired concentration in the middle box, the higher concentration in the upper left-hand corner, and lower concentration in the lower left-hand corner. The process begins in the lower left-hand corner and moves towards the upper right-hand corner. The difference between the number in the lower left hand corner and that in the middle box goes in the upper right-hand corner. Then, the difference between the upper left corner and the number in the middle is put in the lower right-hand corner. On the right, the number represents the parts of the concentration on the left that are used to make the needed concentration. By using proportion math, the volume of each can be calculated.

A figure and an example follow:

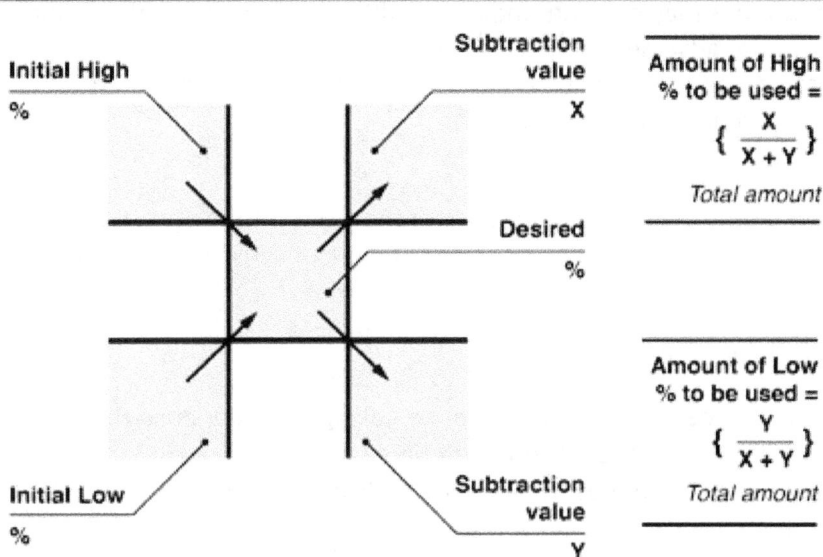

For example, how many grams of 1% hydrocortisone cream should be mixed with an appropriate quantity of 2.5% hydrocortisone cream to make 250 grams of 1.5% hydrocortisone cream?

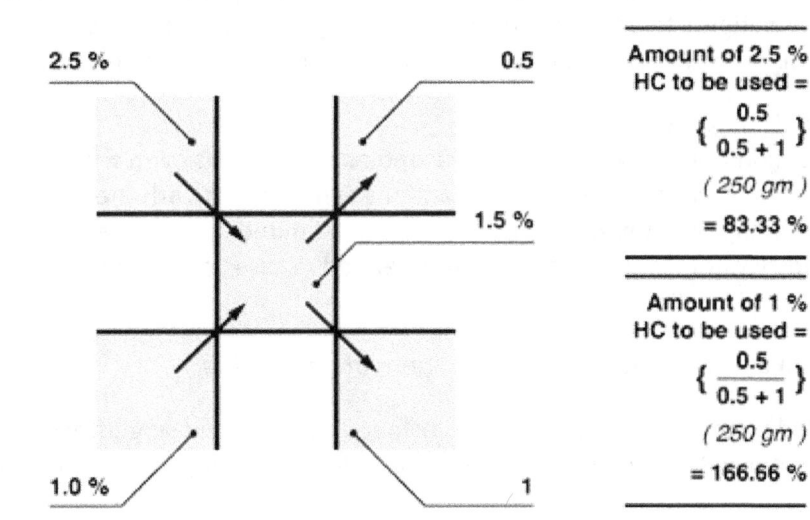

Adverse Effects, Allergies, and Therapeutic Contraindications Associated with Medications

Patient's Medical History
To prevent possible adverse effects with medications, the following information should be included in a patient's medical history:

- All prescription medications, OTC drugs, and dietary supplements taken by the patient
- Chronic and acute medical conditions
- Patterns of prescription compliance

- Allergies to substances, medications, and foods
- Possible interactions that have previously occurred (drug-drug, drug-food, drug-disease etc.)

With access to a patient's medical history, the pharmacist can determine if there are any risks to the patient. Certain medications may be contraindicated with particular medical conditions or health concerns. Allergies or prior adverse reactions to one medication may also impose an allergy risk to other medications in the same class. A complete medical history helps the pharmacist prevent drug interactions and serious clinical consequences.

Compliance
Compliance with a medication refers to adherence of the patient to the prescribed medication as directed by the prescriber. Non-compliance is one of the major causes for discontinuation of a medication.

The following are examples of non-compliance:

- Not taking the full dose of the medication, i.e. taking a smaller dose than what was prescribed
- Not taking medication for the full length of time (stopping early)
- Not adhering to the time of day to take the medication (i.e. night vs. morning)
- Discontinuation of treatment
- Taking expired medications

Non-compliance with a medication can impose significant harm to the patient. There are many reasons for non-compliance, such as physical issues, cognitive problems, misunderstandings, and fear of or experience with side effects. Pharmacies have systems to help keep track of refills and reminders (calls, texts, and emails) for patients to promote compliance. The physician's office can send notifications to the patient and his or her physician when the patient is not compliant with treatment.

Common and Severe Side (or Adverse) Effects
An adverse drug reaction is a reaction that is undesirable, yet happens even when a medication is taken according to its standard dosing. Adverse drug reactions can manifest with the first dosing of the medication or can develop over time. They can happen in a limited area of the body (locally), or can affect the whole body (systemic). An intervention is needed in cases of serious adverse drug reactions that can cause injury and fatality.

The different types of adverse reactions to medications are as follows:

- Compounded pharmacologic effects that include tolerance and side effects
- Peculiar and unpredictable effects (idiosyncratic drug reaction, which could be life-threatening)
- Chronic effects
- Delayed effects
- Effects at the end of treatment
- Treatment failure
- Genetic reactions

Allergies
The following are symptoms that indicate an allergy to a medication:

- Hives
- Skin redness and rashes or other types of reactions

- Swelling in the face, throat, tongue or other area of the body
- Difficulty breathing, wheezing, or chest tightness
- Irregular or rapid heartbeat

Severe form of these reactions can indicate an anaphylactic reaction, which is life-threatening and requires immediate emergency treatment. Emergency Medical Services (9-11) should be contacted right away in cases of suspected anaphylactic reactions to any substance. It is common for patients to confuse allergic reactions and adverse events. Therefore, it is important for the pharmacy staff to ask about the symptoms a patient experiences, so that the reaction can be categorized correctly.

Allergy with Foods and Excipients
There are some medications and supplements that contain food-based ingredients, and therefore, precautions need to be taken when prescribing such substances to a patient with food allergies. The coatings of medications, for example, can have excipients such as lactose, maltodextrin, and other starches that can cause allergic reactions in a person susceptible to those ingredients. Other medications, including Prometrium (a hormone medication), contain peanut oil so patients with peanut allergies should avoid such formulations. Some calcium products and omega-3 supplements are derived from shellfish; hence, a person with a seafood allergy may need to avoid these supplements. Patients with dietary restrictions, such as celiac disease or gluten intolerance, should avoid capsules made with gluten fillers or gelatin. If there are any questions about the ingredients, it is best to contact the manufacturer.

Therapeutic Contraindications Associated with Medications
Alcohol
Alcohol should be avoided while patients are on prescription medications. Consumption of alcohol with medications can cause nausea, vomiting, fainting, loss of coordination, or extreme drowsiness. More severe reactions can lead to heart problems, internal bleeding, and difficulty breathing. Certain medications, when combined with alcohol, can cause toxicity. As alcohol is a strong CNS depressant, combining it with other depressants, like benzodiazepines or sleeping medications, can be dangerous and can cause respiratory failure. If alcohol is combined with a high dose of acetaminophen, there is potential for serious liver damage. Additionally, if alcohol is consumed while taking metronidazole, the patient can experience significant side effects including nausea, vomiting, abdominal pain, cramps, facial redness, headache, tachycardia, and liver damage.

Age
Age has a significant effect on the pharmacology of medications. Maturation during childhood causes various changes in body composition, accompanying growth and development. Therefore, newborns, infants, children, and adolescents often do not receive full adult dosages. As mentioned, medication doses should be appropriately calculated based on the age and weight of the child. There are many medications that are not approved by the FDA for children and yet are used "off label." Unexpected reactions can happen when medications are not studied in pediatric populations. For example, tetracycline is contraindicated in children because it can bind with the calcium in bones, modify bone cartilage, and cause growth retardation. Generally, if a physician prescribes a medication that is not approved for use in children, pharmacy technicians should consult with the pharmacist, who will rely on their professional judgment about how to proceed (i.e. dispense the medication or talk with the physician).

In elderly adults, there can also be significant changes in pharmacokinetics and pharmacodynamics of a medication. Geriatric populations often have comorbid conditions, including cardiovascular disease, diabetes, and renal insufficiencies. Aging can decrease the body's clearance of a medication, resulting in buildup and manifesting in unwanted effects. Routine blood work and dose adjustments may be necessary in the geriatric population.

OTC Medications

Some OTC medications impose significant risks with certain disease conditions. A few OTC medications can lead to an increase in blood pressure, so these may be contraindicated in patients with hypertension. The following medications are known to cause problems for patients with hypertension:

- NSAIDS (ibuprofen and naproxen)
- Decongestants like pseudoephedrine
- Migraine formulations with caffeine.

Patients with high blood pressure should talk to a pharmacist or a physician before taking OTC medications or herbal supplements.

Pregnancy

During pregnancy, medications should be prescribed carefully, to prevent harm to the developing fetus. For some medications, there might not be enough data available regarding safety during pregnancy, and therefore, must be used cautiously after weighing the benefits versus the risks. Many medications are contraindicated during pregnancy, as they have teratogenic effects and can cause birth defects. If a patient is on a teratogenic medication prior to pregnancy, the medication should be stopped upon conception. A few examples of medications that are contraindicated in pregnancy include ACE inhibitors (e.g. ramipril, enalapril, lisinopril, etc.), ARBs (losartan, candesartan, irbesartan, etc.), isotretinoin, tetracycline antibiotics, hormonal therapies, and immunosuppressants (e.g. methotrexate).

Dosage and Indication of Legend Drugs, OTC Medications, and Herbal and Dietary Supplements

Dosage and Indication of Legends

Legend drugs are those that require a prescription. The following information is required to be on prescription labels as mandated by the Food, Drug, and Cosmetic Act:

- The name and address of the pharmacy dispensing the medication
- The prescription number
- The date the prescription was filled
- The last date for refills
- The name of the prescriber
- The patient's name
- The instructions for use
- Any precautions or things to not take while on the medication

OTC Medications and Dietary Supplements

Some medications are available "over the counter," or OTC, without a prescription. OTC medications are still regulated by the FDA, as the manufacturing and sales of these medications are regulated under the Federal Food, Drug, and Cosmetic Act. There are some medications that are classified as OTC, yet, due to federal or local laws, require pharmacy staff to intervene with patients buying the medication. The patient needs to sign a ledger before the sale can be completed. Examples include medications with pseudoephedrine or emergency contraceptives.

Dietary supplements, unlike OTC medications, are not regulated by the FDA. *The Dietary Health and Supplement Act of 1994* defines the guidelines that dietary supplements must meet, including those that:

- Contain a vitamin, mineral, herb, botanical, and/or amino acid
- Are sold as a capsule, tablet, powder or liquid
- Are not purposefully marked to be the sole source of nutrition
- Has the labeling "dietary supplement"

OTC Medications Ingredients

OTC medications often contain various ingredients, especially those intended to treat coughs, colds, and flu. It is important to cross-check the ingredients to prevent duplication of treatment. Two medications that pose a risk for overdose are acetaminophen and dextromethorphan, which are commonly used in cough and cold preparations such as Theraflu and Nyquil. Moreover, OTC sleep aids often have identical ingredients found in antihistamines. It is, therefore, important to check the ingredients in OTC medications to prevent duplicate therapies. The pharmacist should help the patient to pick appropriate OTC medications and counsel them accordingly.

Dosage of Acetaminophen

The maximum daily dose of acetaminophen is 4,000 mg for people with a healthy liver. For those with compromised liver function, the maximum dose is only 2,000 mg per day. In some cases, people with liver disease cannot take acetaminophen at all. As acetaminophen is metabolized primarily in the liver, it is important to follow the dosing instructions to prevent liver damage. Consumption of excessive acetaminophen causes saturation of liver enzymes and buildup of acetaminophen. The metabolic by-products of acetaminophen damage liver cells (hepatocytes).

Dosage of Controlled Substances

The following are the usual range of dosages, available forms, and routes of administration for controlled substances:

- Hydrocodone/acetaminophen: There are two dosage components: the hydrocodone can range in strength from 2.5 mg to 10 mg, and the acetaminophen can range from 325 mg to 650 mg. Depending on the severity of pain, doses are either one or two tablets, as needed for pain. It is important not to exceed 4000 mg of acetaminophen each day with the dosing. The medicine is available in oral tablets of different strengths and as an oral solution.

- Lorazepam: This drug is usually taken PRN or as needed, with up to a total of 6 mg each day in divided doses. This medication is available in two forms: oral tablet and injectable solution.

- Methylphenidate: This drug can be dosed up to 72 mg each day. Immediate release tablets can be taken once or twice a day, while extended-release formulations are only taken once a day. This medication is available in two forms: oral tablets and oral extended-release tablets.

Dosages for Antibiotics
The following are the usual ranges for dosing and available forms for antibiotics:

- Amoxicillin: Usually dosed at 250 mg to 500 mg every 8 hours, or at a higher dose (500 to 875 mg) every 12 hours. This drug is available in a chewable tablet, a capsule, and a powder to make suspensions.

- Penicillin VK: This drug is usually dosed at 125 mg to 500 mg every 6-8 hours. It is available in either oral tablets or a powder to make suspensions.

- Cephalexin: The dose of this drug is 250 mg to 500 mg every 6 to 8 hours. It is available as oral capsules and powder for oral suspensions.

- Cefuroxime: The dose of this drug is usually 250 mg to 500 mg every 12 hours. The forms available are tablets and a powder for oral suspensions.

- Azithromycin: This drug can be taken in multiple combinations; the possibilities are as follows: a single dose of 1000 mg, 500 mg for three days, or one dose of 500 mg followed by four days of 250 mg. This drug is available either in oral tablets or a powder for oral suspensions.

Dosages for Antidepressants
The following are the typical dosages, form, and routes of administration for antidepressants:

- Amitriptyline: This medication can be started at a dose of 10 mg and can be increased to up to 300 mg per day. The dose can be taken at one time or divided over 2-3 occurrences. This drug comes in oral tablets and intramuscular injections.

- Bupropion: The usual daily adult dose for this drug is 150 mg to 300 mg, either in divided doses or in a single extended-release tablet. The maximum daily dose is 450 mg. This drug is available in standard or extended-release tablets.

- Citalopram: This drug is dosed at 20 mg to 40 mg daily; it is recommended not to exceed 40 mg per day. Citalopram can be taken in oral tablets or as an oral solution.

- Mirtazapine: This drug is usually dosed between 15 mg to 45 mg each day. It is available either in regular oral tablets or disintegrating oral tablets.

Dosage of Antihypertensive Medications
The usual dosage range, forms, and routes of administration of common antihypertensive medications are outlined below:

- Hydrochlorothiazide (HCTZ): The dosage for HCTZ can range from 25 mg to 100 mg per day, which can be taken once or in divided doses throughout the day. This medication is available as tablets, capsules, and as a solution.

- Atenolol: Based on the medical conditions, the usual dose of atenolol is 25 mg to 100 mg daily, with a maximum daily dose of 200 mg. This medication is available in oral tablets and as IV injections.

- Amlodipine: This drug can be prescribed from 2.5 mg to a maximum of 10 mg each day and is available as an oral tablet.

- Losartan: This medication is usually prescribed at 25 mg to 100 mg each day, and can be taken all at once or divided into two doses. This drug is available as an oral tablet.

Practice Questions

1. What is the correct interpretation of the following prescription directions: "1 capsule qid"?
    a. Take one capsule every other day
    b. Take one capsule at night
    c. Take one capsule four times a day
    d. Take one capsule three times a day

2. If the adult dosage for amoxicillin is 500 mg, what would be the appropriate dose for an infant that is 6 months old and what is the name of the formula used for infant dosages?
    a. 20 mg, Fried's Rule
    b. 1.67 mg, Fried's Rule
    c. 500 mg, Young's Rule
    d. 20 mg, Clark's Rule

3. Which of the following medications should not be combined with Warfarin?
    I. Aspirin
    II. Diclofenac
    III. Celecoxib
    a. I and II
    b. I and III
    c. II and III
    d. All of the above

4. Which of the following medications should not be taken in combination with nitroglycerin and what would be the result if they were taken together?
    a. Warfarin, excessive blood thinning
    b. Sildenafil, irreversible hypotension
    c. Allegra®, increased heart rate
    d. Sertraline, increased depression

5. If a patient is receiving chemotherapy, which of the following is likely to be prescribed to help with side effects?
    a. Anti-histamines
    b. Propranolol
    c. Promethazine
    d. Nitroglycerin

6. How many 400 mg tablets are needed to make 1 liter of a 1:250 solution?
    a. 30 tablets
    b. 10 tablets
    c. 4 tablets
    d. 400 tablets

7. How many tablespoons are in 4 ounces?
    a. 8
    b. 22
    c. 1
    d. 120

8. What type of dosage form is dissolved under the tongue?
    a. Buccal
    b. Inhalation
    c. Subcutaneous
    d. Sublingual

9. Why is important to collect the patient's medical history before filling a prescription?
    a. It is not usually important, unless the patient is elderly.
    b. It can provide an allergy history and prevent dangerous drug reactions.
    c. It can help the pharmacist predict the next medical condition.
    d. It can make it easier to provide refills.

10. A patient has brought in a prescription for Diazepam. Which of the following conditions is the most likely reason that the patient needs this prescription?
    a. Hypertension
    b. ADHD
    c. Epilepsy
    d. Depression

11. A drug needs to be stored at room temperature (68 °F). What is the equivalent temperature in degrees Celsius?
    a. 36 °C
    b. 72 °C
    c. 68 °C
    d. 20 °C

12. Under what class of controlled substances do some benzodiazepines fall?
    a. Class II
    b. Class I
    c. Class III
    d. Class IV

Answer Explanations

1. C: The abbreviation "qid" means four times a day, hence the other options incorrectly direct how often to take the capsule.

2. A: Fried's Rule is the formula that should be used to calculate dosages for infants and toddlers up to two years old. The 20 mg is found by entering the given values into the formula:

$$Child's\ dose = \frac{Child's\ age \times adult\ dose}{150}$$

The other formulas are not specifically intended for infants and Clark's Rule is based on weight.

3. D: All of the listed medications impose a risk when taken with Warfarin, as they increase the blood-thinning activity and can lead to the blood becoming too thin.

4. B: Sildenafil and nitroglycerin should not be taken together, as both cause blood vessel dilatation, leading to the potential of irreversible hypotension. The other listed combinations do not have documented direct effects when taken in combination with nitroglycerin.

5. C: Promethazine is an anti-emetic, which can help the patient deal with nausea from the chemotherapy. The other drugs would not help with hair loss, nausea, memory problems, weakness, or other side effects associated with chemotherapy.

6. B: Using proportions, one can calculate how many grams of the medication are needed for the solution. Afterwards, the number of grams can be converted to the number of tablets by solving a proportion for the dose in each tablet and the number of grams needed.

7. A: Recalling the conversion of tablespoons to mL, 1 tbsp.= 15 mL, and 1 ounce= 30 mL, so there are 120 mLs in 4 ounces. When divided by 15 mL (equivalent of 1 tbsp), one finds 8 tbsp. = 4 ounces. The other answers are incorrect because they do not apply the conversions correctly.

8. D: Sublingual means under the tongue. Inhalation is through the nose or the mouth. Subcutaneous is an injection that goes under the skin. Buccal refers to the cheek inside the mouth, but not under the tongue.

9. B: Collecting the patient's history can help identify allergic reactions or drug-drug interactions. Although in some cases having the patient's history can help track which medications may need to be refilled, it's not the primary intent.

10. C: Epilepsy is caused by overactive neuronal signaling in the brain, so a central nervous system depressant can calm such activity. Hypertension, ADHD, and depression do not improve with this type of medication and potentially, it can be harmful.

11. D: The correct answer of 20 °C can be found using the appropriate temperature conversion formula:

$$°C = (°F - 32) \times \frac{5}{9}$$

12. D: Some benzodiazepines fall under Class IV of controlled substances. These are highly addictive, both physically and psychologically, so they are typically not prescribed for long-term use.

Pharmacy Law and Regulations

Material Safety Data Sheets (MSDS)

These forms are available as a book or online; each pharmacy should have a book that can be quickly accessed in the event of an accident. It is an OSHA requirement to have a MSDS book in every pharmacy. The MSDS pages contain information about the materials and chemical compounds, including identifying physical features and what should be done in the case of a spill (i.e. precautions and procedures).

There are ten sections to the MSDS. The starred ones are particularly helpful to know:

- Product Identification (Section I)
- Name of Manufacturer and contact information*
- Active Ingredients (Section II)
- Active ingredients and the lethal dose (50)
- Physical and Chemical Data (Section III)
- Fire and Explosion Data (Section IV)
- Flammability*
- Hazardous combustion products*
- Reactivity Data (Section V)
- Conditions for Chemical Instability
- Toxicological Properties (Section VI)
- Route of entry and hazards*
- First aid statements*
- Carcinogenicity*
- Effects of Chronic Exposure
- Ecological Data (Section VII)
- Aquatic Toxicity
- Preventative Measures (Section VIII)
- Types of protective equipment (gloves, eye, respiratory, other) *
- Waste Disposal*
- Storage and Handling requirements*
- First Aid (Section IX)
- What to do if exposed*
- Preparation information (Section X)
- Date MSDS was prepared
- Who prepared MSDS/contact information*

Hazardous Waste in Pharmacies

Pharmacies produce a variety of hazardous waste products, which necessitate proper disposal. Some of these items include the following:

- Expired medications

- Incorrectly compounded medications

- Items that have been contaminated with bodily fluids
- Equipment (not machine, but attachable items) that can be disposed of that was used to dispense or make hazardous materials
- Chemotherapy drugs

Storage of Hazardous Substances and Waste
There should be a designated bin for hazardous waste, specifically designed for such collection. The waste should be stored in the hazardous waste bin until it is picked up by an outside company for disposal.

Handling Hazardous Substances and Waste
Hazardous items should be handled with care and placed in bags that are marked with symbols identifying them as hazardous or biohazards.

Disposal of Hazardous Substances and Waste
There are outside companies that will come to the pharmacy to pick up hazardous waste that is generated.

Prevention and Treatment of Exposure to Hazardous Substances

Eye Wash Station
If a medication or chemical splashes into the eye, it is important to thoroughly flush the eye to remove the splashed substance. Individuals who wear contact lenses should remove the lenses promptly upon exposure. Some pharmacies will have an eye wash station, which requires the assistance of another person to help turn it on. While allowing the water to flush steadily over the eyes for at least 15 minutes, another person should call for emergency assistance.

If there is not an emergency eye wash station at the pharmacy, normal saline should be used to flush the eyes and the individual should receive emergency medical care.

Exposure to Skin
To prevent accidental skin exposure to hazardous substances, regular use of personal safety equipment, such as gloves or gowns, is highly recommended.

It is a possibility that while working in a pharmacy with a medication or chemical, skin contact with the substance can occur; if so, a supervisor should be notified immediately. If clothing comes into contact with the hazardous substance, it should be removed and the skin that was exposed to the chemical should be rinsed in cool water for at least 15 minutes.

Accidental skin exposure can result in burns, blisters, rash, hives, irritation, or reddening. For painful areas, a cool damp compress can be applied, unless there is a burn, in which case the area should be covered with a dry sterile dressing. Second or third degree burns require immediate help from medical professionals.

Ingestion of a Hazardous Chemical
Wearing a face mask during the preparation or compounding of medications and keeping food items far away from the pharmacy preparation areas are important for preventing accidental ingestion of hazardous substances.

- If accidental ingestion of a hazardous substance has occurred, supervisors must be immediately notified. Also, emergency medical assistance is needed.

- The MSDS for the identified substance will provide information on indicated treatment.

- Vomiting should only be induced with a product like ipecac syrup if indicated on the MSDS. If the substance is corrosive or if the person is unconscious, vomiting should *NOT* be induced.

Inhalation of a Hazardous Material

In compounding IV medications, powders are needed to properly prepare the medication, which presents a potential to inhale hazardous substances. If inhalation does occur, the supervisor should be notified promptly and the person should be moved into an area with fresh air. It is important to check if the person who inhaled the hazardous substances can still breathe. Emergency medical assistance should be called. To prevent inhalation of hazardous substances, using a face mask while preparing a compound with a powder is recommended. In the event of a spill, airflow can make a difference in preventing the spread of the spill from one area to the entire pharmacy.

Spill Kit

Spill kits are used for small or medium spills in the pharmacy and the location of the kit should be made known to those who are using hazardous materials and chemicals. The spill kit will contain control materials and personal safety equipment; it can be specialized to the area where one is working and to the type of substance being handled.

In the event of a spill, it is important to do the following:

- Follow the pharmacy's detailed spill response plan.

- Notify everyone in the area where the spill occurred and, if needed, evacuate.

- If clothing has been contaminated, remove it. Also, if skin has come into contact with the chemical, make sure to flush the area of skin in accordance to the guidelines above.

- Review the MSDS to find relevant information about the flammability and volatility of the spilled chemical.

- The MSDS should also provide information about what personal safety equipment is needed. With the particular chemical, the recommended safety equipment and respiratory protection should be donned.

- Use the absorption spill kit in the pharmacy for small or medium spills. If a larger spill occurs, it may be necessary to request outside help. Also, it is important to follow local procedures and policies.

- After the spill has been absorbed, place the materials from the spill in chemical spill bags which can then be disposed.

- When appropriate, wash the area of the spill with water and detergent.

- Communicate with the supervisor that a spill has happened.

Controlled Substance Transfer Regulations (DEA)

Drug Enforcement Administration (DEA)
The DEA is a governmental agency set up in 1973 to implement laws around drug use and to fight drug trafficking. The Controlled Substances Act serves as the guiding document. This agency shares jurisdiction with the Federal Bureau of Investigation and with Immigrations and Customs Enforcement.

The DEA focuses on the following objectives:

- Instructing the public, especially through programs in the community targeted at youth, to lower the use of illegal and diverted drugs

- Supporting local and state law enforcement to assist in lowering drug-related crime and fighting/violence

- Disrupting origins and providers of illegal and diverted drugs on a local, national, and international level

Controlled Substances Act (CSA)
The CSA was enacted in 1970 by the U.S. Congress as Title II of the Comprehensive Drug Abuse Prevention and Control Act. Through the CSA, every Federal law relating to the manufacture, regulation, and sale of certain controlled substances (narcotics as well) were made. Also, the CSA allowed for the creation of five controlled drug classes (Schedules I-V) and what criterion warrants the medications in each class. Updates are made to the Act and the drug schedules to reflect up-to-date information and research.

Explanation of Schedules I-V Controlled Drug Classes
Classification is based on currently accepted medical use for treatment and the likelihood of abuse or dependence on the drug.

- *Schedule I Substances*: These drugs do not have accepted medical use in the US, but can be used by researchers who've obtained special permission by the FDA. Examples are heroin, peyote, and methamphetamine (also known as ecstasy).

- *Schedule II Substances*: These drugs have a high risk for abuse with extreme psychological or physical dependence. Examples are narcotics such as morphine, codeine, and fentanyl; stimulants such as amphetamine and methylphenidate; and others such as cocaine, amobarbital, and pentobarbital.

- *Schedule III Substances*: These drugs have less risk for abuse than Schedule I and II drugs, but the potential for abuse is still present and they still pose a risk for psychological or physical dependence. Examples include narcotics that include combination products such as Vicodin® or Tylenol® with Codeine; and non-narcotics such as ketamine, dronabinol, and anabolic steroids.

- *Schedule IV Substances*: These drugs have less risk for abuse compared to substances in Schedule III. Examples are narcotics such as propoxyphene and non-narcotics, such as alprazolam, clonazepam, lorazepam, and midazolam.

- *Schedule V Substances*: These drugs have less risk for abuse compared to substances in Schedule IV. Substances in this class are generally used as cough suppressants, antidiarrheals, and for analgesic purposes. Examples include pregabalin and small amounts of codeine used in cough suppressants.

Transfer of Controlled Substances
Pharmacies are responsible for the physical transfer of controlled substances and for the precision of the inventory and records. For two years after the transfer, the pharmacy must keep the records immediately available for inspection by the DEA.

An outside firm may be hired by the pharmacy to take stock, pack, and coordinate the transfer of its controlled substances to another location (pharmacy, original supplier, or original manufacturer).

Depending on the schedule category of the substance, DEA Form 222 (Schedule II) or other written documentation (Schedule III or IV) containing the drug name, dosage form, strength, quantity, and the date of transfer is filled out.

Controlled Substance Documentation Requirements

Documentation Requirements for Receiving, Ordering, and Returning Controlled Substances
DEA Form 222 must be filled out either electronically or on paper by the pharmacy to order, transfer, or return Schedule II medications. The DEA Form 222 once filled out, needs to be stored so that it can easily be accessed during an inspection if requested (applies to both electronic and paper records). On the DEA Form 222, the date, the name of the medication ordered, and the amount are required.

There are several rules that need to be followed when filling out and filing the DEA Form 222:

- Do not make alterations to the form. If a mistake is made while filling out the form, a new form should be used.

- For paper versions: the green copy of the form is mailed to the local DEA office.

- For paper versions: the brown copy of the form needs to be kept and filed at the pharmacy for at least two years.

Documentation Requirements for Loss/Theft of Controlled Substances
In the event of a loss or theft of any controlled substance at a pharmacy, the procedures outlined below must be carried out within one business day of discovering that theft or loss has occurred.

- Notify the local DEA Diversion Field Office in writing, as the theft of controlled substances is considered a criminal act and a source of deviation, which requires the DEA be notified.

- It is not clearly required by federal law or policies, but it is important to also inform local law enforcement and state regulatory agencies.

- The DEA needs to be informed of the loss/theft precisely, without any intermediaries (i.e. other parts of the corporation) and the notice needs to be signed by an authorized individual of the registrant.

- DEA Form 106 (Report of Theft or Loss of Controlled Substances) must be filled out by the pharmacy. This form will document what happened to lead to this situation and the amount of controlled substances involved. The following information should be included on the form:

- Pharmacy name and address
- DEA registration number
- Local Police Department name and phone number (if the pharmacy has contacted)
- Kind of theft (for example: armed robbery, break-in, etc.)
- Any identifying label features used on the containers (marks, symbols, or price codes)
- Record of which controlled substances are missing, including the strength, dosage form, and size of container or National Drug code numbers

If the reported lost/stolen material is found after filing and notifying local authorities and the DEA, a written notification must be given to clear up why no Form 106 was filed after the initial notification.

<u>Formula to Verify the Validity of a Prescriber's DEA Number</u>
The formula is very specific for DEA numbers. In order to test the legitimacy of a DEA number, the following requirements must be met:

- DEA numbers have two letters accompanied by six numbers and a "check" number.
- The type of registrant is identified by the first letter in the DEA number. This could be *M* for a mid-level practitioner or *P/R* for manufacturer/researcher.
- The second letter in the DEA number represents the first letter of the registrant's last name.
- The sum of the first, third, and fifth numbers is SUM1.
- The sum of the second, fourth, and sixth numbers is SUM2.
- SUM2 multiplied by two is PROD2.
- The last digit in the result of adding SUM1 and PROD2 should be the same as the check number.

Record Keeping, Documentation, and Record Retention

<u>Record Keeping</u>
The pharmacy is required to maintain a log or file of dispensed prescriptions. Each prescription needs to be kept for a minimum of two years. The authorities or Board of Pharmacy needs to be able to review and inspect the log or file of records at any time.

The log or records of dispensed medications should contain the following information:

- Date the medication was dispensed
- Details of the prescription: drug name, strength, and dosage form
- The patient's name
- The quantity of medication dispensed
- The patient's address

It is important to note that Schedule II medication prescriptions need to have their own file, and Schedule III-V prescriptions need to have their own separate files as well. Additional prescription medications that are not controlled substances should also have their own file.

Documentation for Prescriptions and Inventory
In order to be considered legal and valid, all controlled substance prescriptions must contain the following information:

- Patient's full name and address
- The date the prescription was written
- Prescriber's DEA number, name, and address
- Name, dosage form, and strength of the prescribed drug
- Prescribed quantity
- Directions for taking the medication
- The number of authorized refills, if any
- Signature of the prescriber (handwritten for paper version or e-signature if sent electronically)

If any of the above information is missing, the prescriber needs to be contacted by the pharmacist to resolve the information. If a signature is missing on the prescription for a controlled substance, it must be returned for a handwritten signature. However, if the prescription is not for a controlled substance, the prescriber can provide verbal approval via telephone for the missing signature.

Allowed changes to a Schedule II prescription from the prescriber to the pharmacist over the phone include:

- Dosage form, can change from capsule to tablet or vice versa
- Medication strength
- Amount of the medication prescribed
- Directions for taking the medication

The following changes are *NOT* permitted via telephone, even if requested by the doctor:

- Patient's name (spelling, other changes)
- A different controlled substance from what was originally prescribed
- Prescriber's signature, if not previously included

If any of these changes are required, the patient must take the prescription back to the prescriber to obtain the new, corrected prescription.

Verbal or Faxed Orders for Schedule II Medication
In order for a Schedule II medication prescription to be faxed, the patient must meet one of the following specific requirements:

- Resides in a long-term care facility
- Resides in community-based care
- Participating in a hospice program as a patient
- Receiver of compounded home infusion or IV pain therapy

The signature of the prescriber must be on the faxed prescription and the fax will serve as the reported prescription document.

Only in emergency situations are verbal orders for Schedule II medications recognized. The quantity of medication dispensed is confined to the amount needed in the emergency situation. Within seven days of the emergency verbal order, a written prescription for the amount dispensed must be mailed or delivered to the pharmacy.

Inventory of Schedule II Medications

A continuous log inventory must be kept for Schedule II medications; this log will manually track when each pill is dispensed. Each quarter, the manual inventory needs to be reviewed and compared line-by-line with the pharmacy's electronic inventory system. This inventory is separate from the log of other medications. Schedule II prescriptions also should be filled at a separate time or counter from other prescriptions and returned to their secure storage area; these drugs should never be left out in the open.

Record Retention

Paper prescriptions must be kept on file for two years. Electronic logs/inventory must be stored permanently. The other retention requirements for all of the various types of records used in a pharmacy can be found in credible published pharmacy journals, websites, and informational venues.

Restricted Drug Programs and Related Prescription-Processing Requirements

Thalidomide

The program S.T.E.P.S. (System for Thalidomide Education and Prescribing Safety) is used for patients that are prescribed Thalidomide. Mandatory counseling, pregnancy testing (if applicable), and registration are required before patients can receive their first prescription. Continued regular pregnancy screenings and counseling are required for patients before refills can be dispensed.

Isotretinoin

The iPledge program is used to confine drug distribution. Before patients can receive their first prescription, they must register for the program, undergo pregnancy testing (if applicable), choose two types of birth control, and promise to keep all scheduled appointments. In order to refill subsequent prescriptions, female patients need to take monthly pregnancy tests, use the iPledge system to describe her methods of birth control, and answer questions about the iPledge program.

Clozapine

This prescription medication requires using a program to track the patient's white blood cell count and the absolute neutrophil count. There are different programs through each manufacturer; any of these programs are acceptable, as long as the pharmacist and prescriber can have access to the files to see how the patient is reacting to the medication.

How to Identify a Forged Prescription

Individuals who falsify or change prescriptions frequently make common mistakes that are easy to recognize. It is important to review new prescriptions for these "tell signs" or mistakes:

- Personal information on the prescription is conflicting.

- The type of doctor who "wrote" the prescription would not usually prescribe the specified type of medication, for example, certain specialists or cardiologists. This "tell sign" could hint that the prescription blanks were stolen.

- Mistakes in the dosing instructions or abbreviations are hints, such as an unusual dose for the specified medication or mistakes using the codes.

- Glaring changes on quantity to be dispensed or number of refills. Sometimes erasing happens by the prescriber, but in such cases, the prescriber should be contacted to confirm the numbers.

- Varying types of ink on the prescription can indicate that changes have been made to a previously valid prescription.

- Usually no refills are provided on Schedule II prescriptions; if there are refills requested, check with the prescriber to make sure it was not in error.

- Observe the quantity prescribed closely.

Mailing a Prescription

There are certain pharmacies that provide mail service to patients for their prescriptions. Regulations for which medications can be mailed differ from state to state, so it is important to check local laws before sending medications. In order to make sure the prescriptions arrive safely, a special cushioned envelope should be used for mailing and cotton should be used to pack the pill bottle to cushion the medication and minimize the chance of breaking the bottle. To prevent confusion, patients should be notified that their medications are being mailed in cases where the pharmacy or patient are unaccustomed to mailed prescriptions.

Professional Standards Related to Data Integrity, Security, and Confidentiality

Data Integrity
To keep track of product quality, safety, efficacy, purity, and compliance, it is mandatory in the regulated healthcare industry that required data is recorded and reported. Patients and healthcare professionals are dependent on a strong record of traceable data. It is important to enter data accurately and attribute any information changes to a person on a certain date and time. The data must be available for review and inspection over the lifetime of the record. Complete and consistent records are essential to ensure the integrity of the data.

Privacy Rule of HIPAA
The Privacy Rule of HIPAA took effect on April 14, 2003 and was the first exhaustive federal rule created to shield protected health information (PHI). This rule requires that pharmacies that electronically keep track of patient information or complete financial and administrative transactions comply with HIPAA.

Security Rule of HIPAA
These requirements were put in place on April 20, 2005. The security standards set administrative, physical, and technical protections that the pharmacist must take into account to safeguard the confidentiality, integrity, and availability of PHI. While all PHI is covered, the requirements are designed to particularly address PHI at risk through the potential of unauthorized access and interception during electronic transmission. As with the privacy rule, any pharmacy that sends health information electronically needs to follow the security rule.

Health Insurance Portability and Accountability Act (HIPAA)

This Act was put in place in 1996 and took effect in 2003, with the goal of ensuring patient's medical information does not get incorrectly distributed. Healthcare professionals are required by HIPAA policies to do the following:

- A designated privacy officer must be employed by the healthcare company
- Create a system to correctly secure protected information
- Develop and maintain HIPAA-compliant privacy policies
- Inform patients of their rights under HIPAA and how they can obtain their health information
- Inform patients what to do if they experience a privacy violation
- Instruct employees how to correctly ensure patient privacy
- Penalize employees who do not correctly follow HIPAA policies and procedures

Medication Preparation

Maintaining confidentiality is a high priority in patient care. During medication preparation, it may be necessary to discuss the medication or provide the pharmacist with more information about the patient. Although the location of the pharmacy may not make it easy to see the patients in the waiting room, it is highly likely that they can still hear what is being said. It is essential to remember to use a quiet voice when discussing patient and prescription information in a location where other people can overhear. If a loud voice is used and other people hear the information, it is a serious violation of HIPAA and can cause embarrassment for the patient as well as distrust in the pharmacy.

Identifiable Patient Information

Identifiable patient information consists of any information that could be used to identify the patient, including:

- Patient's name
- Patient's ID number
- Patient's address
- Patient's phone number
- Patient's Social Security number

Any conversations that include identifiable patient information should take place in the most confidential setting possible. For paperwork with this information, precautions should be taken to keep the paperwork and information out of sight from other patients or people that do not have a justifiable reason to see it. For information that is stored on a computer, the screen must be turned so that it is not readable or visible to other patients or the public. Additionally, computers should be password-protected and locked when they are not in use.

Releasing Confidential Patient Information

Conditions for releasing confidential patient information are as follows:

- If other providers who are involved in the patient's treatment need the information to correctly coordinate patient care

- Other parties, medical and otherwise, can obtain information if the patient has signed a release of information

- In order to receive correct payment, information can be released to a third-party payer

- Request by the patient for their own use through a signed release of information
- Public Health Officials in the case of certain infectious diseases or dog bites because the information can be considered to pose a threat to public health
- In certain situations, by subpoena

<u>Backing Up and Archiving Data</u>
Pharmacy application service providers should back up files daily. Also, in order to prevent loss of records during a natural disaster, fire, or system failure, it is recommended that the back-up copies of the data are stored at another location.

Requirement for Consultation

The Omnibus Budget Reconciliation Act of 1990 amended the Federal Medicaid Act and set standards for filling and distributing prescription medications. This act requires each state to have a Prospective Drug Use Review (DUR) program, making sure that pharmacists document important information about the drug and present this orally and through written documentation to the patient.

Consultation with patients can be affected by several factors such as the patient's literacy level of and his or her language spoken and understood. Notes about the patient's language can be recorded in the notes section. In the case of prison inmates, phone calls can be used for consultations but in general, with all patients, it is preferable to carry out the consultation in person.

FDA's Recall Classification

There are three classes of recalls (Class I, II, and III) that the Food and Drug Administration (FDA) uses to systematically address the severity of the recall:

- Class I is the most serious recall; drugs that fall under this class present risks for serious adverse health conditions or death.
- Class II is slightly less serious than Class I; drugs that fall under this class are unlikely to cause serious adverse health conditions or death, but the drugs can lead to temporary health problems.
- Class III is the least serious recall; this type is used when an FDA regulation has been violated but adverse health conditions are not likely to occur.

FDA Market Recalls are another type of warning issued for a drug, where minor violations need to be corrected or the drug needs to be removed from the market. Medical device recalls are part of FDA Medical Device Safety Alerts.

<u>Food and Drug Administration (FDA)</u>
The FDA was formed in 1927 to provide oversight for the production and safety of food and drugs in the United States. The main goal of the FDA is to safeguard and advance public health by overseeing and modulating the production of the following products:

- Food products
- Prescription medications
- Over-the-counter medications

- Tobacco products
- Dietary supplements
- Biological drug products
- Vaccines
- Blood transfusions
- Medical devices
- Cosmetics

The President appoints the director of the FDA, who is also the Commissioner of Food and Drugs. The FDA can examine and implement laws related to food and drug safety through the Office of Criminal Investigations. A majority of the laws that are of interest to, and affect, the operations of the FDA are found in the Food, Drug, and Cosmetic Act.

Federal Food, Drug, and Cosmetic Act (FD&C)
This act was put in place in 1938 after over 100 people died from taking a medication that had traces of diethylene glycol. As technology and manufacturing have evolved over the years, the Act continues to be amended to reflect current standards. This act gives the FDA supervision of the safety of the food, drug, and cosmetic industries.

There are 20 chapters to the FD&C Act, which contain sections on:

- Definitions
- Prohibitions and penalties
- Food adulteration, including bottled water
- Drugs, as well as homeopathic preparations
- Medical devices
- Cosmetics
- Imports and Exports

Infection Control Standards

Antimicrobial Resistance
Antimicrobial resistance is a major issue in hospitals and can lead to patients leaving with infections unrelated to the condition they were originally admitted for. As a result of this problem, it is essential to take preventative measures, such as hand washing, wearing personal protective equipment, employing contact precautions, and antibiotic rotations.

Occupational Safety and Health Administration (OSHA)
Under OSHA, employers are liable for keeping a safe and healthy work environment. OSHA sets standards for maintaining healthy and safe workplaces, and will provide relevant training, education, and outreach to employers.

United States Pharmacopeia and National Formulary (USP-NF)
These are published together in an arrangement called the USP-NF. All medications, including prescriptions and over-the-counter drugs, in the United States must comply with the standards set in the USP-NF. Also, the USP creates standards for food products and dietary supplements. The USP will pass down information to practitioners and pharmacists about medications, along with aspects of drug use. For example, this process is used by the Medicare Prescription Drug Benefit plans to create formularies. Other countries have decided to use the U.S.'s USP, rather than creating their own.

USP 795
This publication applies to non-sterile preparations for compounded formulas that are dispensed to humans or animals.

USP 797
This is a publication that was produced by the United States Pharmacopeia to improve the safety products produced in a compounding environment. It is required by some boards of pharmacy at the state level and recommended by others. It provides guidance on state-of-the-art compounding environments that are sterile and keep patients safe.

Compounding and Manufacturing Medications
The difference between compounding and manufacturing as defined by the FDA is as follows: Compounding is the preparation of patient-specific doses of medications that are prescribed by a physician. Manufacturing is bulk preparation of non-patient specific medications. Pharmacies are legally allowed to compound, but are not allowed to manufacture.

The following are ways that pharmacies violate the law when compounding drugs:

- In anticipation of prescriptions, the drug is made ahead of time
- Use of ingredients that have been withdrawn from the market
- Use of ingredients that are not approved by the FDA
- Commercial scale manufacturing or testing equipment is used in the process
- Reselling to a third-party

Laminar Air Flow
The recommendations by OSHA for biological safety cabinets are as follows:

- Biological Safety Cabinets (BSC) need to be used during the preparation of hazardous medications

- BSCs that vent to the outside are urged (Class II, type B, or Class III)

- Horizontal BSCs are not recommended for putting together hazardous drugs because they increase the chance of drug exposure

Hazardous drugs should not be stocked, unpacked, compounded or handled in an area that has positive pressure relative to the surrounding areas.

Hand Washing
Hand washing is considered the single best preventive measure to stop the spread of hospital-acquired infection. Between each direct patient encounter, a physician's or pharmacist's hands need to be washed (whether with soap and water or alcohol-based rubs). It is important to note that antiseptic hand rubs do not work consistently against spore-forming bacteria.

Record Keeping for Repackaged and Recalled Products and Supplies

Repackaging Log
A repacking log should be maintained in the pharmacy to keep track of the new information for the repackaged drug product. The following must be on the label for repackaged drug products: generic drug name, drug strength, dosage form, name of manufacturer and lot number, and expiration date.

Records for Recalled Products and Supplies
The following must be entered into inventory records for drugs that are recalled or returned:

- Date that the product was removed from inventory
- Identifying information for the product
- Name, strength, dosage form, and quantity of drug removed
- Manufacturer of the product
- Lot or ID number
- The reason the drug was removed from inventory (i.e. recall by manufacturer)
- Initials of technician and supervising pharmacist
- Any other information as required by pharmacy policy

Poison Prevention Packaging Act
This Act was put in place in 1970. Before this time, household poisonings were one of the principle causes of death in young children. The purpose of the Act was to combat and decrease these poisonings. The Consumer Products Safety Commission was empowered by the Act to develop rules about packaging for products that would be applied in households with young children. As a result of the Act, the development and mandatory use of child-resistant caps was instituted, as well as regular safety tests for caps, to ensure standards are met to keep children safe.

Consumer Products Safety Commission
This commission was created by the approval of the Consumer Products Safety Act in 1970, primarily to keep the public safe by reducing avoidable risks with manufactured products. Drugs are not regulated by this agency, but the containers in which that medications are sold fall within the realm of this agency's oversight. The Consumer Products Safety Commission performs research on products that have had numerous or concerning consumer complaints and will issue a recall when needed or prohibit a product that is thought to be dangerous. Consumer complaints about possible dangerous products can be submitted through the agency's toll free number or website.

The Joint Commission (TJC)
This is a non-profit, independent organization in the United States that certifies and attributes achievements to healthcare organizations, such as hospitals. Receiving accreditation from TJC is regarded as the standard for best care in the U.S. Overall, the TJC aims to guarantee that the best possible healthcare is provided to all patients at all facilities throughout the country. Regular reviews and checks of healthcare facilities (including pharmacies) allows for continued success in meeting the goal of the TJC. If a facility does not meet the standards set forth by the TJC, it must follow the recommendations provided within a certain timeframe, and then be reassessed.

Disposing of Medications
Medications need to be properly disposed; the FDA recommends the following to adhere to safe procedures:

- Medications should not be flushed down the toilet unless the package explicitly says to do so.
- Community take-back programs should be used if they are offered in the area.
- The label should be destroyed or made illegible before the medication is thrown away.

- If medications are thrown in the garbage, the following should be done before doing so:
    - Medications should be removed from the original containers and mixed with a substance (coffee grounds or cat litter) and
    - Medications should be placed in a sealed bag or another empty container to avoid leakage.

DEA Take-Back Program

This program is a national event where pharmacies, community partners, and law enforcement agencies support collection sites where community members can return expired or unnecessary medications for proper disposal. After collection, the medications requiring disposal are retrieved by a local DEA representative. The main purpose of this program is to reduce the number of drugs that could possibly be used by unintended persons and to reduce risks to consumer safety by stopping the consumption of expired medication. Also, these events deter improper medication disposal and reduce possible environmental contamination.

Professional Standards of Pharmacy Professionals

General Duties of a Certified Pharmacy Technician

There are many tasks that certified pharmacy technicians are accountable for in retail pharmacies including:

- Taking prescription orders from patients
- Reviewing the electronic system and faxes for prescription orders
- Preparing orders with pharmacy software
- Counting or measuring the proper materials to prepare the medication order
- Keeping patient profiles correct and up-to-date
- Entering insurance claims and making inquiries about continuing insurance issues
- Checking out customers at the cash register
- Managing the pharmacy's stock and inventory
- Responding to phone calls

Under no circumstances should pharmacy technicians provide medical advice to patients. It is essential for pharmacy technicians to maintain current awareness of medications and healthcare information. This equips them to be better able to recognize possible mistakes and other issues so they can notify the pharmacist.

Work Environment at the Pharmacy

There are different types of pharmacy settings where certified pharmacy technicians are employed including:

- Retail pharmacy stores (for example Walgreens, CVS, etc.)
- Hospitals
- Long-term care housing
- Pharmacies specializing in mail orders
- Stores specializing in medical supplies

There are a variety of hours that pharmacy technicians may work, depending on their employer; some technicians work regular 9 am to 5 pm shifts on the weekdays, whereas others may have varying shifts working for 24 hour pharmacies (such as in a hospital or retail). Weekends and holidays are also part of the work schedule, so pharmacy technicians need to keep this in mind. There are professional unions for pharmacy technicians that many individuals choose to join.

Legal Ratio of Pharmacy Technicians to Pharmacists
There are laws at the state level about the precise ratio of technicians to pharmacists allowed at any time. These laws vary between states, and some states' laws will provide the specified ratio, whereas others will simply suggest a ratio. The ratio is often 2:1 or 3:1 for pharmacy technicians to pharmacists. Ideally, limiting the ratio can assure that the pharmacist has enough supervisory capacity and that prescriptions and prepared medications are fully verified before being dispensed.

General Tasks in a Hospital of a Certified Pharmacy Technician
A hospital-based pharmacy technician will likely engage in the following tasks:

- Caring for and ordering stock, certifying inventory, removing expired stock, and putting together returns

- Following and maintaining narcotic inventory

- Making IV and other sterile mixtures, along with chemotherapy and parenteral nutrition, under the supervision of a pharmacist

- Choosing the right medication to fill orders

- Assembling medications for dispensing throughout the hospital

- If local law allows, reviewing other technician's work

- Distributing medications throughout the hospital on a scheduled and on-demand basis to units and nursing floors

- Upkeeping the medication delivery systems, such as to automated dispensing devices

- Keeping patient records accurate and up-to-date

- Keeping the pharmacy clean and in good operating order

- Helping with the training of new technicians

Dispensing of Medication
In most hospitals, the nursing station is the central point of each section. This is where nurses stop for information and obtain instructions for their day. It is common for automatic dispensing devices to also be located at the nursing station. Additionally, in hospitals that have pneumatic tube systems, there is usually a tube stop at each nurse's station. Pharmacy technicians will load the dispensing device or send individual doses through the tubes. The medications will be retrieved and dispensed by the nurses according to doctor's instructions. It is essential that nurses follow the same storage policies for medications as the pharmacy does. Sometimes training will be provided to make sure the rules are being followed uniformly throughout the hospital. In some cases, pharmacy technicians will be sent to check the area to ensure the medications are stored in compliance with law and hospital policy.

Appropriate Clothing for Technicians/Dress Codes

Pharmacies often specific dress requirements for their technicians. For example, at retail pharmacies, business casual clothing is often required, whereas at hospitals, scrubs are often required. The environment of the business—be it more professional or more concerned with safety and cleanliness—often dictates the dress code. The following stipulations may be required, depending on where the technician is employed:

- Scrubs (generally cotton shirt and pants in different colors)
- Foot covers
- Hair bonnets
- Masks
- Protective eyewear such as goggles or other eye coverings

All shoes worn in a pharmacy environment are required to have a closed toe; this is very important for safety when working with chemicals and sharps (such as needles and syringes) as well as for sanitary reasons.

Reconciliation Between State and Federal Laws and Regulations
- State laws and rules can be different depending on which state the pharmacy is in
- Pharmacy law follows the strictest requirements if state and federal law differ

State Board of Pharmacy

There is a board of pharmacy in each state. As a part of the state's Department of Health, the board of pharmacy is responsible for licensing pharmacies, pharmacists, and technicians. Responsibilities are different from state to state. The main purpose is to advance public health and safety through making sure every pharmacy in the state is performing with the same set of high standards. Inspections are carried out by the state board of pharmacy and grades are provided to make sure pharmacies are meeting the set standards. By acting as a go-between, the board can make communication easier between the public, pharmacies, and state governmental agencies.

National Associations of the Boards of Pharmacy (NABP)

This organization is focused on providing assistance and support to the individual state boards of pharmacy. The NABP is meant to stay unbiased and to help maintain uniform standards across the states. Also, the NABP assists with the transfer of pharmacist's licenses across state lines. Founded in 1904, this organization's fundamental purpose is to encourage and preserve public safety. Finally, the NABP administers examinations to evaluate a pharmacist's competence.

Updates on Pharmacy Law

Updates to state and federal pharmacy laws occur often. The following sources help provide the most up-to-date pharmacy law information:

- DEA website: www.dea.gov

- Website for own state's board of pharmacy

- The National Pharmacy Technician Association website and newsletter, see: www.pharmacytechnician.org

- Magazines about pharmacy, such as *Drug Topics*, *Rx Times*, *U.S. Pharmacist*, and *Pharmacy Times*

These updates are also important for a certified pharmacy technician's continuing education hours, as one hour of the twenty required annual hours must be in pharmacy law to maintain certification.

Facility, Equipment, and Supply Requirements

Orange Book: "Approved Drug Products with Therapeutic Equivalence and Evaluations"
There should be a copy of this book accessible in every pharmacy, even though there is an online format available on the FDA's website. The *Orange Book* contains the safety and efficacy information on all products that the FDA has approved. The book contains medications from after 1938, and the first book was published in 1980.

The book classifies medication by:

- Active ingredient
- Proprietary name
- Applicant
- Application number

Reference Materials
- *Remington's Pharmaceutical* provides useful information for compounding medications because it contains the physical characteristics of different drugs and recipes.

- *Handbook of OTC Drugs* provides information on all over-the-counter drugs on the market, along with active drugs as well as inactive ingredients.

- *Drug Listing Act* gives a unique and permanent drug code to every medication, NCD, which labels the manufacturer and size or type of packaging.

Cleaning Items and Equipment Used to Count Medication
Throughout the pharmacy, there are tools and equipment used in the preparation of medications (measuring, counting and pouring) that become dirty or tainted with dust from the medications. At least once a day, these tools and equipment (counting trays and spatulas, etc.) should be washed with hot soapy water. It is also recommended to keep cleaning wipes readily accessible to wipe down counting trays throughout the day. Most pharmacies have separate tools for preparing prescriptions that are often known to cause allergies (sulfa antibiotics and penicillin are examples). In theory, the powder from these medications can be transferred to other medications if counted on the same trays and equipment, leading to an allergic reaction. Any tools used to pour or scoop liquid and cream medications should be cleaned directly after use.

Areas of the Pharmacy to be Cleaned Each Day
Pharmacy Technicians are responsible for keeping the pharmacy as clean as possible on a daily basis. In order to keep the pharmacy clean, dusting should be performed regularly. Below are the daily cleaning tasks that a pharmacy technician should perform:

- Washing off the counter and all surface areas
- Rinsing all tools from medication dispensing
- Washing off keyboards and all phone surfaces
- Taking out the trash from the pharmacy
- Cleaning the floor of the pharmacy using a broom or a vacuum

- Using a wet mop with disinfectant on the pharmacy floor
- Disinfecting the waiting area or lobby of the pharmacy

Practice Questions

1. The following is a DEA registrants number: BJ6125341. What is the check digit and is the number valid?
    a. 1 and yes
    b. 4 and yes
    c. 1 and no
    d. 4 and no

2. Pharmacy technicians have many tasks in the pharmacy. Which of the following is NOT a legal task for them to perform?
    a. Answering phones
    b. Providing medical advice to a patient
    c. Processing orders using pharmacy software
    d. Being on alert for potential errors and notifying the pharmacist

3. Which of the following is a sign that a prescription might be forged?
    a. The number of refills appears to have been altered
    b. The patient is a first-time customer of the pharmacy
    c. No refills are given for a Schedule II medication
    d. The prescription is phoned in by the physician

4. What is needed to order Schedule II narcotics from a wholesale warehouse?
    a. Approval from the FDA
    b. A prescription from a physician
    c. Form 222 must be filled out on paper or electronically
    d. The perpetual inventory shows the Schedule II narcotics are fully stocked

5. When the laws differ between the state and federal level, which laws should be followed?
    a. The most lenient law should be followed
    b. Both sets of laws should be followed to the fullest extent possible
    c. Neither set of laws should be followed because they are different
    d. The strictest law should be followed

6. Which Act below designates five controlled drug classes (Schedules I-V) and specifies the type of medications that are controlled under each class?
    a. Prescription Drug Marketing Act
    b. Controlled Substances Act
    c. Federal Food, Drug, and Cosmetic Act
    d. Poison Prevention Packaging Act

7. How long should dispensed prescriptions be kept on file and should Schedule II prescriptions be kept with other medications that have been dispensed?
    a. Forever; keep everything together
    b. 2 years; keep Schedule II prescriptions separate from other medications
    c. 5 years; keep Schedule II prescriptions separate from other medications
    d. After the prescription is filled; it can be thrown away and there are no prescriptions on file

8. Which of the following is required to follow the Health Insurance Portability and Accountability Act (HIPAA)?
   I. Train employees how to correctly maintain patient privacy
   II. Quietly discuss patient & prescription information so no one in the waiting room can hear
   III. Computer screens with this information must be password-protected and not visible to others
   a. I and II
   b. I and III
   c. II and III
   d. I, II, and III

9. Which of the following explains why separate spatulas and counting trays should be used for medications that are likely to cause allergies?
   a. Each medication should have its own spatula and counting tray
   b. Separate tools are not required, but frequent washing is needed for these medications
   c. The powders of potentially allergen-inducing medications can cross-contaminate other prescriptions
   d. It is unrealistic to keep track of which spatula and counting tray was used for a particular medicine, but pharmacists and technicians should be careful about contamination

10. Which agency is responsible for child-resistant packaging?
    a. DEA
    b. FDA
    c. The Joint Commission
    d. Consumer Products Safety Commission

11. What is the difference between the Orange Book and the MSDS?
    a. They are the same reference materials but both should be kept in every pharmacy
    b. Neither should be contained in the pharmacy, but they differ in the information they contain about medications and chemicals
    c. The Orange Book catalogs all products approved by the FDA whereas the MSDS is the safety information from the manufacturer about the chemical
    d. Neither of these documents is important in a pharmacy

Answer Explanations

1. A: Applying the DEA number formula, the individual should find the check digit and validate it is the same. The formula is to add digits 1,3, and 5 which is SUM1, and then add digits 2,4, and 6, which is SUM2. Then, SUM2 is multiplied by 2, resulting in Product 1. Next, SUM1 and Product 1 are added together. The check digit is the second digit in the answer.

2. B: Certified Pharmacy Technicians are not allowed to provide medical advice to patients; this falls outside of their scope of practice. They are asked to do all of the other tasks listed as options in the answer bank.

3. A: It's possible that the doctor made a mistake or changed their mind when writing the number of refills; however, it's still suspicious if the number of refills has been altered. You should contact the physician by looking up the number to their office (rather than using the number on the prescription pad), and ask them to confirm the number of refills they are prescribing. People must be a first-time customer of a pharmacy at some point, and people often relocate, so it's not necessarily suspicious. Schedule II medications typically do not have refills associated with the prescription. In emergency situations, a physician can call in a prescription as a verbal order, which must then be followed up with a paper version within seven days.

4. C: Form 222 from the DEA must be filled out on paper or electronically to order Schedule II medications from a wholesale warehouse, to transfer Schedule II medications between locations, or to return Schedule II medications to the wholesaler. Approval from the FDA is required for a medication to be marketed. A prescription from the physician is required for the patient to obtain the medication. The perpetual inventory needs to be maintained at all times. However, if all of the Schedule II medications are fully stocked, it is unlikely that the pharmacy will need to order more.

5. D: The strictest law should be followed. If the state has more requirements than the federal government, then the state laws and requirements should be followed. Due diligence should be given to understanding both state and federal laws pertaining to the pharmacy and, if there are questions, follow-up with the appropriate agencies and authorities is required.

6. B: The Controlled Substances Act classifies drugs into five controlled categories. The Prescription Drug Marketing Act ensures that all drugs marketed to the public are safe and effective and do not introduce risk from alterations. The Federal Food, Drug, and Cosmetic Act grants the FDA oversight of the safety of the food, drug, and cosmetic industries. The Poison Prevention Packaging Act requires the use of child-resistant caps on medication bottles.

7. B: Prescriptions should be kept on file for a minimum of two years and Schedule II medication prescriptions must be filed separately from other prescriptions. All prescriptions that were filled, need to be readily accessible during an inspection or visit from authorities. The other answer options are not correct due to 1) not maintaining the prescription file for appropriate length of time, 2) not separating controlled substance prescriptions from regular prescriptions, and 3) discarding the prescription after it has been filled.

8. D: To comply with HIPPA policies, all of the provided choices must be followed.

9. C: It is essential to keep track of tools that were used to dispense medications that could potentially lead to allergic reactions and to only use the tools to dispense the particular medication (i.e. penicillin).

Powders from medications can easily get on other pills that are being dispensed with the same tools. The best practice is to wipe down the tools after use and to mark tools used for certain medications that have higher allergen potentials.

10. D: The Consumer Products Safety Commission is an agency that conducts research on products that are worrisome and also on the latest in child-resistant packaging. The DEA is responsible for enforcing laws related to drug use and illegal drug sales. The FDA is responsible for overseeing drug and food production and the safety of these products in the U.S. The Joint Commission is an agency responsible for determining if a hospital has met the standards for healthcare.

11. C: The *Orange Book* contains all the products the FDA has approved since 1938 and contains the following information about each medication: active ingredient, proprietary name, applicant, and application number. The MSDS is provided by the manufacturer and contains important health and safety information about the referenced chemical. The other answers are incorrect because both the *Orange Book* and MSDS information should be easily accessible in every pharmacy and these reference materials provide different types of information from one another.

Sterile & Non-Sterile Compounding

Introduction

Pharmaceutical compounding refers to the formulation of a product in a pharmacy, distinct from one supplied by a commercial manufacturer, in order to meet the unique needs of a patient as specified by the physician. The reasons for pharmaceutical compounding vary:

- The product might not be available commercially.

- The product may be in short supply (e.g., a product on back-order).

- There may be a change in the dosage form (e.g., formulation of a liquid dosage form from solid tablets or capsules).

- The patient may have an allergy to an excipient (filler) in a product.

- There may be a need for large-scale intravenous or parenteral medications for hospital supply.

- There may be a need to improve compliance by altering the taste and texture of an otherwise unfavorable formulation.

Certain considerations should be considered to ensure the safety and efficacy of a pharmaceutical admixture:

- *Personnel*: It is crucial to delegate the responsibility of compounding a formulation to a person who has the requisite knowledge and expertise in pharmaceutical compounding. If a pharmacy is unable to compound an item, the patient should be referred to another pharmacy that has the ability to formulate it as specified. The designated personnel should have adequate knowledge in the following areas:

- Physical and chemical properties of the ingredients
- Physical and chemical compatibilities between ingredients and excipients (fillers)
- Pharmaceutical calculations
- Use of appropriate methods
- Use of appropriate equipment

- *Premises and environment*: Compounding should be performed in a designated area that ensures an appropriate environment in terms of space, storage, and lighting. The assigned area for compounding should be clean, orderly, and sanitary. The compounding area might maintain a written protocol addressing various issues, such as hand washing, equipment cleaning, and managing staff injuries that result from compounding. The compounding area should have access to water for cleaning hands, equipment, floor, and surfaces.

- *Equipment and supplies*: The pharmacy should have appropriate equipment and supplies in order to formulate pharmaceutical admixtures per the specified standards. Equipment should be routinely cleaned and kept dry to minimize contamination with the formulation ingredients and extraneous materials. Pharmaceutical compounding generally requires the following equipment and auxiliary supplies, in addition to therapeutic ingredients, to formulate a compound:

- Class A prescription balance or analytical balance to weigh the ingredients
- Weighing papers, wax papers, or measuring boats
- Spatula to transfer ingredients
- Mortar and pestle for grinding and mixing
- Graduated cylinders (10 ml and 100 ml)
- Ointment slab
- Cream or ointment base
- Wetting or levigating agent to reduce particle size
- Personal protective equipment (PPE)

- *Resources*: A compounding pharmacy should have adequate resources available to render the intended service. The pharmacist should gather information from peer-reviewed sources, such as academic journals, to formulate a product. If the formula is not available for the intended preparation, it should be prepared utilizing the knowledge of physical and chemical properties of the ingredients, pharmacology, and pharmaceutical science.

Infection Control

In a pharmaceutical compounding practice, personnel are accountable for providing safe and ethical services to patients by strictly following the guidelines of infection control. It is recommended that all personnel adhere to the current infection control programs.

The infection control guidelines should be practiced in the following terms:

- Personal safety and prevention of spreading disease
- Prevention of an infection spread caused from compounding tools and equipment
- Prevention of an infection spread from materials and sources in the compounding environment

To prevent infections, the following routine practices must be employed:

- Hand washing or hand hygiene
- Use of additional barrier precautions, i.e., use of Personal Protective Equipment (PPE)
- Appropriate handling of workplace equipment
- Cleaning of the premises, equipment, and environment
- Appropriate method for handling waste
- Personal care for disease prevention, e.g., immunization

<u>Hand Washing</u>
Hand washing is the simplest and most cost-effective means of preventing the spread of infections. Bar or liquid soaps are recommended for routine hand washing. Antiseptic gels, rinses, and rubs can also be used. The most common antimicrobial agents used in healthcare practices for hand washing are alcohol (70-90%), aqueous chlorhexidine (2% or 4%) solutions, and iodine compounds.

Following the standard, proper, hand washing technique is important in preventing the spread of infection and should include the following steps:

8. 1. Remove rings, watches and other jewelry.

9. 2. Wet hands with warm water.
10. 3. Apply soap or disinfectant preparation.
11. 4. Vigorously rub all areas of hands including the back of hands, palms, fingers, nails and wrists.
12. 5. Continue rubbing for at least 10 to 20 seconds (time varies according to different guidelines).
13. 6. Rinse hands and dry properly using a paper towel.
14. 7. Turn off the tap with the paper towel used to dry hands, and discard the towel.
15. 8. After drying, apply lotions to keep hands moist and healthy.

Standard Hand Washing Technique

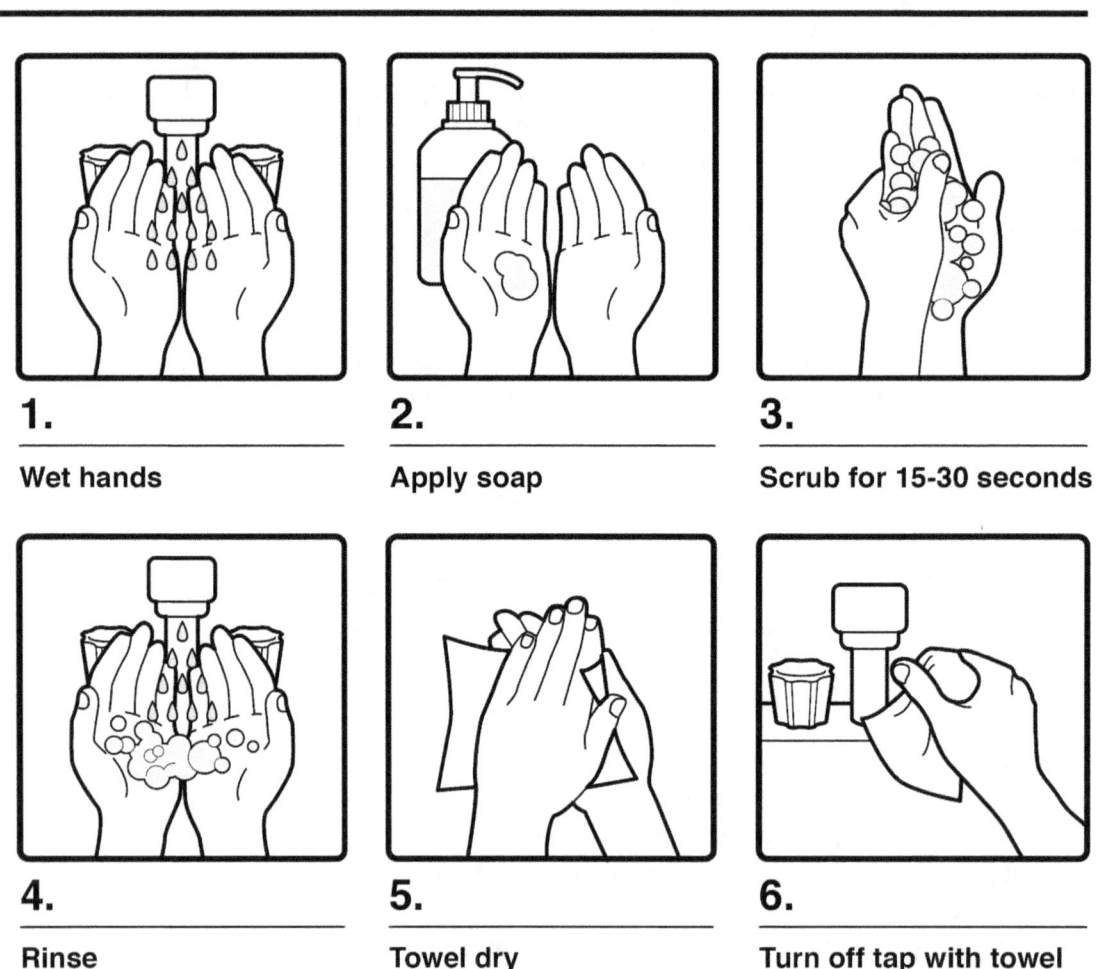

1. Wet hands
2. Apply soap
3. Scrub for 15-30 seconds
4. Rinse
5. Towel dry
6. Turn off tap with towel

Personal Protective Equipment (PPE)
The pharmacy staff should use PPE appropriate to the nature of the contaminating agents. The PPE most commonly used in healthcare facilities are gloves, masks, gowns, head covers, shoe covers, and eye protection. Note that the use of PPE does not eliminate the need for proper hand washing. When used properly, PPE can significantly reduce the risk of infection spread; however, PPE cannot completely eliminate the risk. Staff should never share PPE. PPE should be completely changed after a task, and

used PPE should be disposed of appropriately. Hand washing should be done every time after disposal of the PPE and before attending to another duty.

Gloves are routinely used in compounding practice to prevent contamination and the spread of infection. Their use also helps personnel reduce contamination while performing procedures.

The following considerations should be kept in mind for best use of gloves in practice:

- Gloves should be removed carefully to prevent skin contamination.
- Hands should be washed each time after removing gloves.
- Single-use gloves should not be reused and should be discarded.
- Gloves should be changed after contact with contaminated items, such as linens or wastes.
- Gloves should be purchased from manufacturers that meet the regulatory board standards.

Masks provide respiratory protection from airborne solid particles and droplets. *Droplets* refers to liquid particles larger than 5μm in size. Droplets do not stay suspended in air for very long. and instead fall on various surfaces. N-95 masks are widely used in health practice. The "N" means "not resistant to oil" and "95" indicates that it has 95% efficacy for filtering particles of 0.3 μm size. The National Institute for Occupational Safety and Health (NIOSH) in the U.S. certified that N-95 masks provide adequate protection against airborne particles, but not against gas or vapor. They also provide little protection against direct liquid splashes.

The following considerations need to be considered for proper use of masks in practice:

- Gloves should be removed first, and hands should be washed prior to removing the mask.

- The mask should be removed carefully to prevent contamination to airway or skin.

- Hold the mask, remove ties, and pull mask away from the face. Do not drag the mask over the face.

- Discard gloves and mask, and wash hands afterward.

Infection Control of Environment and Equipment

Environmental surfaces should be cleaned daily and when visibly dirty. These surfaces generally need a low level of disinfectant similar to general housekeeping. The places requiring cleaning include tables, counter tops, floors, bathrooms, doorknobs, sinks, and waiting room chairs. Disinfectants used in daily cleaning are toxic and hazardous and, therefore, should be properly labeled, handled, and stored. The most common disinfectants include alcohols, 3% hydrogen peroxide-based products, phenolic compounds, and household bleach.

The type of disinfectants to be used for cleaning tools and equipment depends on the purpose and level of disinfection required. Here are some examples of routinely-used disinfectants in clinical practice:

- Low-level disinfectants
- Phenolic compounds
- Quaternary ammonium compounds
- 3% hydrogen peroxide
- Hypochlorite household bleach
- Intermediate-level disinfectants

- Alcohols (70-90%)
- Hypochlorite household bleach
- Iodines and iodophor (e.g. povidone-iodine)
- Boiling item for more than 20 minutes
- Ortho-phthalaldehyde
- Glutaraldehyde for 20 minutes
- 6% hydrogen peroxide soak for 5 minutes
- High-level disinfectants
- Boiling item for more than 20 min
- Ortho-phthalaldehyde
- Glutaraldehyde for 20 min
- 6% hydrogen peroxide soak for 5 min
- Sterilization
- Exposure to steam at a high temperature and pressure (autoclave)
- Glutaraldehyde for 10 hours
- Gas sterilization (ethylene oxide)
- Dry heat sterilization

Handling and Disposal Requirements

The ingredients used in formulations should be handled cautiously in order to prevent contamination and degradation. Materials from the same container can be reused until they reach the expiration date labeled on the container. Staff should make sure to decrease exposure to the remaining content each time any material is withdrawn from the container.

The withdrawal of ingredients from the container should be performed by a trained individual who has expertise in handling the materials. If an ingredient is transferred from the original container to a different container, the new container should be labeled with the necessary information including name, supplier, lot number, and expiration date.

The pharmaceutical waste generated during compounding should be appropriately handled and disposed. In the past, pharmacies used to destroy waste materials by incinerating them, washing them down a sink or toilet, or returning them to the sales representative/manufacturer. However, incineration pollutes the air, and dumping medications down a sink or toilet causes environmental pollution. Many medications are hydrophilic, biologically-active, and resistant to wastewater treatment. Therefore, disposal of pharmaceutical waste must comply with the corresponding state and federal regulations, as well as those regulations specified by the U.S. Environmental Protection Agency (EPA). A compounding pharmacy may contact a third party that has expertise in pharmaceutical waste collection, handling, and disposal.

There are three types of waste produced in a pharmacy:

- *Solid waste*: all solid, liquid, and gaseous waste

- *Hazardous waste*: any substance or combination of substances that could produce harmful effects on the health and safety of a person

- *Infectious waste*: blood, bodily fluids, blood products, sharps that are infectious, and waste from the laboratory

Waste receptacles are waste-specific. There is usually a specified container for biohazards and sharps (including infectious sharps); it is typically a red/dark orange receptacle that is labeled "bio-hazard."

For pharmaceuticals (expired or unused non-hazardous drugs), there are separate disposal containers (typically dark blue); these containers are appropriate for disposal of items such as antibiotics, IVs, and ibuprofen. For hazardous drugs, there are typically waste bags with the label "Hazardous Drug Waste"; these are leak-proof and come in a variety of colors, with the exception of white.

Documentation

Documentation helps in systematically tracing, evaluating, and replicating the steps that were involved in a compounding process. Compounding pharmacies should maintain four sets of records:

16. Master formulation records

- Official name, strength, and dosage form of the compounded product
- Calculations used to determine and check quantities of components and doses
- Description of all ingredients and the individual quantities
- Compatibility and stability information (including available references)
- The equipment used/needed to make the preparation (when relevant)
- Instructions for mixing
- Order the ingredients were mixed
- Temperature during mixing or other environmental settings
- Amount of time of mixing
- Other relevant factors for repeating the preparation as compounded
- Sample label information, including legally required information as well as the following:
- The generic name and the amount of each active ingredient
- The Beyond Use Date (BUD) that was given
- Required storage conditions
- The number for the prescription
- The container that was used to dispense the product
- Requirements for packaging and storage of the product
- Final preparation description
- Procedures used for quality control and expected results

17. *Compounding records* describe what happens while the formulation is being compounded
18. *Standard operating procedures* (SOPs), including equipment maintenance records
19. *Ingredients' records,* including Certificates of Analysis (C of A) and Material Safety Data Sheets

Documentation should be preserved for the period of time specified by state laws. Records should be available in the pharmacy during the retention period for auditing purposes. Proper documentation is important to ensure consistency in batch-to-batch preparations. Records of complaints by patients and of serious harmful events due to compounded medications should be kept on record for at least two years from the day the prescription was dispensed. Follow-up investigations on the complaints should be included in the records. Calculations of the quantity of each component in the compounded medication should also be documented. The types of calculations that are necessary for compounding were previously described.

Master Formulation Record (Compound Formula)

Name of compound: _____

Strength: _____ Dosage form: _____ Total quantity: _____

Ingredients	Manufacturer	DIN	Quantity

Preparation instructions: _____

_____

_____

_____

Prepared by: _____

Reference: _____

Compounding Record

```
                    Affix Rx label              Source of formula: _____
     Compound name: _____              Beyond-use date: _____
     Strength: _____                   Deviation from master formula: ____
     Dosage form: _____                _____
     Quantity: _____                   _____
     Batch: _____                      Deviation approved by: _____
     Date prepared: _____
```

Ingredients	MFR	DIN	Lot #	EXP date	Quantity	Measured by	Verified by

Calculation: _____

_____

_____

Calculated by: _____ Verified by: _____

Formulation prepared by: _____

Signing off (Pharmacist): _____

Determination of Product Stability

Prior to dispensing any formulation to a patient, it is important to ensure the accuracy and completeness of the formulation by reviewing each step of the compounding.

In the *preparatory steps*, the following criteria should be met:

- The ingredients, excipients, and equipment are appropriately selected for the formulation.
- The calculation of each of the ingredients and excipients is correct.
- The formulation ingredients are accurately measured.
- The formulation meets the requirements of intended use and ensures stability.

In the *final formulation*, the following criteria need to be met to ensure accuracy and stability:

- The actual yield is consistent with the calculated yield.

- The *physical properties* (e.g., color, odor, consistency, clarity) of the final formulation are consistent with what was predicted. Alteration in physical properties is an indicator of incompatibility.

- The formulation should be suitably labeled. The label should meet all legal requirements, and must include the *discard after date* or *beyond-use date*.

It is recommended that samples of the formulations are sent to an analytical testing laboratory (or this can be done within the pharmacy) to assess the stability of the formulation over the storage period.

Analytical testing aims to assess the following:

- Physical characteristics (color, odor, consistency, taste, etc.)
- Homogeneity
- Concentration
- pH
- Sterility
- Nonpyrogenicity
- Expiration date and beyond-use date

During compounding, personnel should avoid ingredients and conditions that could result in a sub-potent formulation. Adequate knowledge about chemical reactions helps in ascertaining product stability and degradation over the period of compounding, dispensing, and storage.

Commercially-available pharmaceuticals carry an expiration date based on the stability data. The *expiration date* refers to the calculated timeframe within which a product retains its physical and chemical stability and therapeutic efficacy, based on a published monograph.

The *beyond-use date* refers to the date after which a compounded preparation should not be used and should be discarded. A beyond-use date should be assigned conservatively, utilizing professional judgement, and applying knowledge from pharmaceutical science and compounding experience. The beyond-use date should never be later than the expiration date of any of the ingredients.

These factors must be considered when specifying a beyond-use date:

- The chemical nature of the drug and its degradation kinetics
- The formulation dosage form and the ingredients
- Any possible microbial growth
- The packaging container
- The storage conditions
- The intended length of therapy
- Any information obtained from suppliers and published literature

In absence of stability information, the beyond-use date could be specified as illustrated in the following table:

Beyond-use Date by the Type of Formulation	
Non-aqueous formulations	Not later than the time remaining until the earliest expiration date of any of the ingredients or 6 months
Aqueous oral formulations	Not later than 14 days since compounded and when stored at controlled cold temperatures
Aqueous topical/dermal and mucosal liquid and semisolid formulations	Not later than 30 days

Selection and Use of Equipment and Supplies

The following considerations should be considered when selecting tools and equipment for compounding practice:

- Equipment and utensils used in pharmaceutical compounding should have a suitable design and capacity that will allow for effective admixing. The type and size of the equipment to be utilized depends on the intended purpose of compounding, the dosage form, and the volume/amount to be compounded.

- The surface of the equipment should be chemically-inert and should not alter the admixture through chemical reaction, addition, or absorption.

- Tools and equipment should be properly stored to avoid contamination and routinely cleaned.

- All electronic, automated, mechanical, and other instruments used in preparing or testing admixtures should be routinely calibrated and inspected.

- The cleaning of equipment should include extra care and caution when the preparation includes cytotoxic agents, antibiotics, and hazardous materials.

- When possible, equipment can be dedicated for a specific job that involves hazardous chemicals or requires high precision. Disposable equipment should be used to reduce the bio-burden and cross-contamination.

- The ingredients used in pharmaceutical compounding should be carefully selected to ensure acceptable strength, quality, purity, and stability in the final formulation. In the selection and use of ingredients, the following measures should be taken:

- The compounding ingredients should be collected primarily from a preferred source that meets United States Pharmacopeia (USP) and National Formulary (NF) grades. If not available, another source that ensures high quality grade, e.g., Analytical Reagent (AR), American Chemical Society (ACS), and/or Food Chemicals Codex (FCC) can be used.

- Components produced in an FDA-registered manufacturing facility should be used first. If that's not possible, the purity and safety of the ingredients should be ensured by reasonable means, which includes obtaining a Certificate of Analysis (C of A), determining the reputation of the manufacturer, and determining the reliability of the source. The C of A should be maintained in record for future reference.

- Pharmaceutical products such as tablets, capsules, and injectables are often used as sources for active ingredients. Staff should make sure that the pharmaceutical products used in compounding are collected from bottles labelled with a batch control number and expiration date.

- If any of the ingredients do not carry an expiration date assigned by the manufacturer, then the container should be labeled with the date of receipt. A conservative expiration date should be assigned, based on the nature of the chemical, its degradation pattern, and the storage condition.

- To ensure safety and avoid toxicity when compounding a formulation for human use, it is important to check that the required medication is not on the FDA list of drugs withdrawn from the market.

- To ensure consistency and quality of the formulation, it is important to receive an ingredient from the same supplier every time. Ingredients from different suppliers may have a variation in physicochemical properties, resulting in an alternative drug response of the final formulation.

- Ingredients and excipients utilized in a particular formulation should be selected based the following criteria:

- Physical properties
- Compatibility
- Patient conditions (allergy, disease state, use of other medications)
- Intended use
- Possible duration of treatment
- Possible drug-drug and drug-excipient interactions
- Route and frequency of administration

Sterile Compounding Processes

The *sterile compounding process* must follow the United States Pharmacopeia 797 terminology and specifications.

- *Sterile compounds* refer to pharmaceutical formulations that are free from all forms of disease causing pathogens and thus, require extra caution during handling, preparation, and storage. They are prepared by utilizing appropriate techniques that eliminate, kill, or deactivate microorganisms including bacteria, fungi, viruses, parasites, and other disease-causing agents.

- *Sterilization* is the process of achieving sterility of a compound, which can be done by utilizing one or more techniques, including heat, irradiation, chemical, or filtration.

- *Asepsis* is the practice of maintaining sterility in products and facilities. The formulations that generally require asepsis include the following:

- Intravenous formulations, including total parenteral nutrition
- Intramuscular medications
- Subcutaneous medications
- Ophthalmic solutions and suspensions
- Chemotherapeutic medications

- If the formulation does not guarantee sterility, it should be discarded, and strategies should be adopted to prevent future errors. Thus, before dispensing sterile medications, the medications should be carefully inspected to check for any *signs of incompatibility* or *contamination*:

- Formation of precipitate
- Presence of particles or unidentified objects in solutions
- Opaque or cloudy solutions, when they should be clear
- Change in color or development of a color that is unanticipated
- Obstacle when withdrawing medication through a needle from the container
- Visible separation of the ingredients

Laminar Flow Hood

A *laminar flow hood* is designed to provide a space in pharmacy that is free of contaminants and particulates for the purpose of compounding sterile preparations. Air from the room is drawn through a High Efficiency Particulate Arresting (HEPA) filter and blown back toward the user to keep a steady stream of filtered air flowing over the items in the hood. Both vertical and horizontal hoods are available, as well as others with different airflow patterns designed for specific uses. The laminar flow hood must be maintained according to manufacturer specifications and cleaned thoroughly before every use to ensure no contaminants are present.

Cleaning the laminar flow hood requires the use of a proper technique:

1. Collect your cleaning equipment: 70% ethanol or other disinfectant, sterile gauze or other laboratory grade wipes.

2. Dress in personal protective equipment, including gloves, mask, goggles, foot coverings, and a gown.

3. Turn the hood on, and allow the hood to run for five minutes.

4. Remove any items that do not belong in the hood.

5. Spray the internal surfaces with the disinfectant, and clean with sterile wipes using a sweeping back and forth motion. Do not spray disinfectant into the HEPA filter.

6. Allow the hood to air dry.

Specifying Beyond-Use Date for Sterile Compounds

Beyond-use dates (BUDs) for sterile compounds should be assigned very conservatively. They must not exceed the earlier of the dates, based on the following two criteria:

- The expiration dates of each of the ingredients, according to their monograph and supplied reference

- Risk of microbial contamination or microbial stability, related to the compounding processes and storage conditions

General Guidelines to Specify the BUD for Sterile Compounds

BUD without additional sterility testing			
Risk of contamination	At controlled room temperature	With storage in refrigerator	With storage in freezer
Low	48 hours	14 days	45 days
Medium	30 hours	9 days	45 days
High	24 hours	3 days	45 days

Non-Sterile Compounding Processes

There are several general considerations to take into account before initiating pharmaceutical compounding (these also apply to sterile compounding):

- The physical and chemical properties of active ingredient(s)

- The pharmaceutical and therapeutic uses of active ingredient(s)

- Analysis of whether the admixture will provide adequate topical or systemic absorption

- Assessment of whether any components of the admixture will render unexpected allergic, toxic, or undesirable reactions

- A dedicated clean and sanitized area is available for compounding

- Compounds are performed one at a time in that dedicated area

- For orally-administered admixtures: an assessment of what the possible effects of gastro-intestinal pH and hepatic metabolism on the bioavailability for active ingredient(s) would be

The *compounding process* (sterile and non-sterile) involves five distinct steps:

1. Preparing

- Review the prescription and determine whether the preparation would be safe and would fulfill the intended purpose.

- Make a list of chemical ingredients and excipients required for the formulation.

- Perform calculations to determine the amount of active ingredients and excipients required to compound the admixture.

- Select suitable equipment, ensuring that it is clean.

- Wash hands and wear appropriate PPE.

- Arrange necessary ingredients and equipment to perform compounding.

2. Compounding

- Perform the admixing according to the formulary and directions in the prescription.
- The admixing should utilize the art and science of pharmaceutical compounding.

3. Checking

- Check certain physical parameters of the admixture, including color, odor, consistency, and pH.
- Enter the information in the compounding log.
- Label the compound.

4. Recording and signing: All information should be entered and signed by a pharmacist, confirming that the assigned procedure was carried out properly (to ensure quality and to serve the intended purpose) as specified in the prescription.

5. Cleaning

- Clean the equipment and compounding areas.
- Dispose of waste and PPE.
- Wash hands.

Techniques Used in Non-Sterile Compounding
- *Blending*: mixing two substances together
- *Communition*: making a substance into small, fine particles
- *Geometric dilution*: mixing two different ingredients together of unequal quantities, starting with the ingredient of smallest quantity and adding the same quantity of the other ingredient (of larger amount), continuing to repeat until all the ingredients are used
- *Levigation*: the use of water or another solvent to carry an insoluble drug powder through the process
- Powder can turn into a thin paste with use of less water
- *Pulverization by intervention*: for powders that do not crush easily, a solvent (usually an alcohol) dissolves the powder can be used to intervene.
- Mixing dissolved powder on an ointment slab or in a mortar helps the solvent evaporate, and the powder will come out in finer particles.

Practice Questions

1. The Class A prescription balance is commonly used in compounding pharmacies. What is the sensitivity of a Class A prescription balance?
    a. 5 mg
    b. 6 mg
    c. 7 mg
    d. 10 mg

2. In a horizontal laminar flow hood, how far should one work from the front edge of the work surface?
    a. At least 4 inches
    b. At least 6 inches
    c. Less than 6 inches
    d. At least 2 inches

3. Which of the following could contribute to infection spread in a compounding pharmacy?
    I. Droplet transmission
    II. Contact transmission
    III. Airborne transmission
    a. I and II
    b. I and III
    c. II and III
    d. I, II, and III

4. How often should a laminar flow hood be certified?
    a. Every 3 months
    b. Every 6 months
    c. Every 9 months
    d. Every 12 months

5. While working in a compounding pharmacy, you notice that a bottle of disinfectant is leaking and spreading all over the floor. When you report to the pharmacist, he asks you to take care of it. What would be the appropriate spill-handling procedure?
    a. Wear gloves and wipe it
    b. Pour some rubbing alcohol on it and wipe it off
    c. Spread paper towels on the spill
    d. Consult MSDS for handing the chemical

6. Which are the following are reasons for compounding?
    I. The patient may have an allergy to an excipient in a product.
    II. There may be a need for large-scale intravenous or parenteral medications for hospital supply.
    III. There may be a change in the commercial insurance coverage
    IV. There may be ways to change the product's taste or texture
    a. I, II, III
    b. I, II, IV
    c. I, III, IV
    d. I, IV only

7. Substances or combination of substances that can produce harmful effects on the health and safety of a person are classified as which type of waste?
    a. Solid waste
    b. Biodetrimental waste
    c. Infectious waste
    d. Hazardous waste

8. What are the four types of records that compounding pharmacies must maintain on file?
    a. Master formulation records, compounding records, standard operating procedures, ingredients' records
    b. Master formulation records, compounding records, sterilization records, ingredients' records
    c. Master formulation records, compounding records, PPE records, ingredients' records
    d. Master formulation records, compounding records, personnel certification records, ingredients' records

Answer Explanations

1. B: The Class A prescription balance can weigh between 120 mg to 120 gm. It has a sensitivity of 6 mg, which means just 6 mg of weight will move the balance pointer one division off the equilibrium (or one degree).

2. B: One should work at least six inches from the front edge of the work surface to ensure adequate sterile compounding and airflow. When the distance is less than 6 inches, the laminar flow air can start mixing with the outside air, which increases the risk of contamination. It is also important to position hands in a way that helps to avoid blocking airflow.

3. D: All of the provided choices are potential causes of transmission. Review section 3.1 for more details about modes of infection spread and strategies to control infection.

4. B: The correct answer is 6 months.

5. D: The MSDS (Material Safety Data Sheet) is a document that carries information about potentially hazardous chemicals and how to handle them safely.

6. B: Pharmaceutical compounding, or the unique formulation of a product in a pharmacy to meet the specific needs of a patient, can occur for a variety of reasons. For example, the product might not be available commercially or it might be on short supply or back-order. Sometimes, there can be changes in the dosage form or patients may have allergies or aversions to fillers or tastes and textures of a product. The pharmacy may be able to make a special formulation to alleviate these issues. There may also be a need for large-scale intravenous or parenteral medications for hospital supply. Insurance coverage should not directly cause a pharmacy to make a special compound in their facility.

7. D: Hazardous waste is any substances or mixture of substances that can produce harmful effects on the health and safety of a person. Solid waste, despite its name, refers to all solid, liquid, and gaseous waste. Infectious waste is all waste that contains blood, bodily fluids, blood products, sharps that are infectious, and waste from the laboratory. Biodetrimental waste is fictitious and not an identified type of pharmaceutical waste.

8. A: Compounding pharmacies must maintain master formulation records, compounding records, standard operating procedures, and ingredients' records. The master formulation records are detailed records of all the compounds made in the pharmacy, requirements for storage, sample labels, instructions for mixing, the equipment used to make the product, etc. Compounding records explain what happens during the formulation's compounding process. Standard operating procedures (SOPs) include equipment maintenance records and detail the general policies and procedures the pharmacy adheres to and ingredients' records, include Certificates of Analysis (C of A) and Material Safety Data Sheets (MSDSs), along with other information from the supplier.

Medication Safety

Introduction

Medication dispensing errors refers to the deviations in a medication dispensed to a patient from that which was written in a prescription order.

An error might fall into one of these categories:

- Incorrect medication
- Incorrect dose
- Incorrect dosage form
- Incorrect quantity
- Incorrect or confusing direction
- Incorrect or inadequate labeling
- Incorrect patient
- Incorrect preparation etc.

Certain situations can increase the chance of medication dispensing errors:

- Unorganized work flow
- Work interruptions and distractions
- Poor handwriting and inadequate/incorrect information on prescriptions
- Excessive workload and stress
- Long shifts (fatigue)
- Ineffective communication with physicians and patients
- Lack of skilled personnel
- Inadequate staffing

Error Prevention Strategies for Data Entry

Medication dispensing errors can be prevented or minimized by adopting systematic approaches in workflow.

20. 1. Collect adequate information about the patient and the prescription.

    a. Verify the patient's information with the information written on the prescription— e.g., name, address, and date of birth. In the case of a patient with hearing or visual impairment, find an alternative means to communicate with the patient to verify the information.

    b. For existing patients, find the patient's profile by entering the patient's date of birth, and then verify by matching two unique identifiers on the pharmacy profile and the prescription.

    c. For new patients, verify two unique identifiers (e.g., date of birth and address) between the prescription and the newly-entered pharmacy profile before entering the prescription.

    d. If any part of the prescription information is missing, incomplete, or unclear, contact the corresponding physician to reconfirm the information.

e. Be cautious when dispensing look-alike or sound-alike drugs. It's important to be careful about zeros, decimal points, and abbreviations.

f. Incorporate an IVR (interactive voice response) that prompts physicians to leave thorough details about the prescription. The message should require that they provide details about the prescriber (prescriber's name, license number, phone number), details about the patient (patient's name, date of birth, phone number), and details about the medication (name, strength, direction of use, duration of treatment, and number of repeats/refills).

g. Verify the "therapeutic use of the medication" with the patient to confirm that the treatment is appropriate for the patient's condition.

h. If a verbal prescription is received through an IVR or direct communication, collect all necessary information and always reconfirm by reading back the prescription.

i. Pharmacy prescription entry load can be reduced through electronic prescriptions.

21. 2. Provide an environment that reinforces accurate prescription entry.

3. Provide supportive measures that assist in accurate information entry for filling out the prescription. Consider integrating the following at the prescription entry/drop-off station/counter:

- A scanner with a re-sizable prescription imaging system on the screen
- A stand to hold the prescription at eye level
- Image magnification and zooming software
- Adequate light and counter space

4. Allow entry of only one patient's prescriptions at a time. Keep other prescriptions away to avoid possible mix-up. Distractions should be reduced as much as possible.

5. Always use "baskets" to keep individual patient's prescriptions separate. This strategy significantly decreases dispensing errors and allows better tracking of patients to be served (in order according to drop-off or requested pick-up time).

6. Provide facilities that allow remote prescription entry during peak hours.

7. Patients should be encouraged to place orders in advance through the IVR, online, or email to reduce the workload at peak hours.

8. The technicians' shifts should be planned efficiently so that adequate staff is available during busy hours (or predicted busy days).

22. 9. Employ additional staff and/or utilize automated processes to identify and correct errors.

a. If feasible, provide additional employees to cross-check the prescription entry before it reaches the pharmacist for the final check.

b. Design the pharmacy software in a way that requires action by the staff to enter a patient's information completely prior to processing the prescription.

c. Keep the hard copy and/or scanned image of the prescription available for the pharmacist for the final check.

Patient Package Insert and Medication Guide Requirements

Written patient information refers to any written information about a prescription medication that is provided to the patient.

There are three categories of written information:

- Patient Package Insert (PPI)
- Medication Guide (MG)
- Instructions for Use (IFU)

The written patient information addresses various issues that are specific to the medication regarding its safe and effective use. It also discusses special directions and precautions to avoid medication-induced adverse events. Not all medications have written patient information. Patients can ask their healthcare provider or pharmacist for details about their prescriptions.

Patient Package Insert (PPI)
PPIs are developed and submitted voluntarily to the FDA by the manufacturer. PPIs are approved by the FDA.

For certain classes of medications, it is mandatory that PPIs be provided to patients—these include oral contraceptives and estrogen-containing products. The FDA warrants the safe and effective use of these products by requiring that patients be fully informed about the benefits and risks associated with the uses of these medications.

Manufacturers also voluntarily submit PPIs for other medications to the FDA for approval; however, distribution of these PPIs to patients is not mandatory.

Medication Guide (MG)
MGs are paper handouts that contain FDA-approved information about specific drugs and drug classes. They are provided in order to help patients avoid adverse events. The manufacturer of the medication develops the MG, and the FDA approves it. The FDA requires that MGs be supplied to patients receiving certain prescribed drugs and biological products. MGs help patients prevent serious adverse effects and make informed decisions (by providing information about serious side effects of a product). They also help patients adhere to the product's directions associated with product's effectiveness.

Instructions for Use (IFU)
IFUs refer to written patient information that is produced by the manufacturer and approved by the FDA. They are provided to ensure proper use of certain medications with complicated dosing instructions.

Issues that Require Pharmacist Intervention

There are certain activities in pharmacy operations that require *pharmacist intervention* in order to ensure safe and effective use of medications by patients. A pharmacist needs to utilize various resources, professional judgement, and/or consultation with the prescriber and patient to make a decision under those circumstances. Provided below are examples of situations where a technician should seek the pharmacist's attention for guidance and the appropriate intervention.

Drug Utilization Review (DUR)

A DUR is an authorized, systematic, and ongoing review about the prescribing, dispensing, and use of a medication in respect to a specific patient's condition(s). It incorporates a comprehensive review of the patient's health history and medication profile for the purpose of making an appropriate decision prior to dispensing a medication.

A pharmacist intervention in a DUR improves the quality of patient care by preventing adverse drug reactions and minimizing inappropriate drug therapies. Pharmacy software generally picks up on various issues that require a DUR intervention. When a DUR conflict arises, the pharmacist needs to use an appropriate intervention code to fill, or reject to fill, the prescription.

Here are some examples:

- *Drug-drug interactions*: patient taking two or more medications that could interact and alter the intended therapeutic effects and/or cause some adverse effects

- *Drug-disease interactions*: patient receives a prescription for a medication that is contraindicated in the patient's disease condition

- *Drug-patient precaution*: medication that could be inappropriate for a patient in respect to the patient's age, gender, allergies, pregnancy, or other factors

- Inappropriate treatment duration

- Medication overuse/misuse/abuse or under-utilization

- Drug dosage modification

- *Formulary substitutions* (e.g., therapeutic interchange, generic substitution)

Scenario for a DUR: A patient is on warfarin as a blood thinner for prevention of cardiovascular events. The patient receives a prescription for naproxen 500 mg (non-steroidal anti-inflammatory medication) for treatment of his tendinitis. This situation will result in a DUR conflict for drug-drug interaction requiring pharmacist intervention. The pharmacist needs to consult with the prescriber to change the therapy as naproxen could augment the effect of warfarin and cause internal hemorrhage (bleeding).

Adverse Drug Event (ADE)

An *ADE* refers to an unwanted effect of a medication that could cause injury to the patient. If untreated, an ADE could lead to organ damage, disability, hospitalization, and even fatality. A pharmacist should appropriately intervene in a situation of an ADE to ensure the best patient outcome.

An ADE can result from augmented pharmacological effects, which are mostly dose-dependent. It is more prevalent with medications that have a narrow therapeutic index (i.e., dose margin). For example, warfarin is an anticoagulant that has a narrow therapeutic index. The dose of warfarin is determined and adjusted based on routine blood work. An augmented effect of warfarin from a high dose or interaction with other medications can cause an ADE, i.e., an internal hemorrhage.

An ADE may also result with a medication for which a patient has medical allergies. For example, a patient allergic to penicillin can experience anaphylactic reactions from amoxicillin.

Over-the-Counter (OTC) Recommendations

Patients often seek *OTC recommendations* for the treatment of minor ailments. However, the pharmacist should assess the patient's condition(s), including the disease and concurrent use of other medications, prior to giving any recommendation. Pharmacist intervention is crucial in OTC recommendations to ensure the patient's safety and benefit. Before recommending an OTC medication, a pharmacist should rule out any alarm symptoms that might require an emergency or physician intervention.

Scenario for OTC Recommendation: A patient comes to the pharmacy counter asking the technician for an OTC pain reliever for his neck and chest pain. When the pharmacist collects the patient's information, the description of his pain (pain radiating to the left side of the body) strongly resembles symptoms of ischemic heart disease. The patient should be immediately referred to a hospital without any OTC medication recommended.

Miscellaneous Interventions

There are certain other situations that require pharmacist intervention. Technicians should be advised to always seek the pharmacist's attention while dealing with these issues:

- *Formulary substitution*: Therapeutic and generic substitutions often require an intervention by the pharmacist for the best treatment outcome. A pharmacist might contact the prescriber if drug-drug/drug-disease interactions or allergies warrant a therapeutic substitution.

- *Misuse/overuse*: Certain medications, including narcotics, controlled substances, stimulants, and psychotomimetic agents, may be misused or overused. A pharmacist should intervene appropriately to limit the use of those medications by the patient. The pharmacist can educate the patient and consult with the prescriber when he or she suspects medication overuse.

- *Missed dose*: Patients often seek advice regarding missed doses. The recommendations for a missing dose vary significantly for different medication types, including maintenance medications (e.g., for hypertension, diabetes), antibiotics, and oral contraceptives. A pharmacist can appropriately intervene in such situations to find solutions and offer the best advice to the patient.

Look-Alike and Sound-Alike (LASA) Medications

Some drug names look like or sound like other drug names. These include both generic and brand names of medications. LASA medications are a common cause of medication errors. With the presence of thousands of medications in the market, errors due to confusing drug names are possible and can be significant.

Consider the following examples:

LASA Medications	
Drug name	Often confused with
amlodipine	aMILoride
acetazolamide	acetoHEXAMIDE
ARIPiprazole	RABEprazole
chlorpropamide	chlorproMAZINE
ClobaZAM	ClonazePAM

Pharmacies can adopt the following strategies to prevent or reduce errors associated with LASA medications:

- Printing both the brand name and the generic name on prescriptions and pharmacy labels
- Adding the indication of each medication on a prescription
- Designing clinic-office/pharmacy software in a way that prevents LASA medications from appearing concurrently
- Changing the appearance of LASA medications to attract attention to their dissimilarities
- Implementing independent double-checks throughout the entire pharmacy workflow
- Storing LASA medications in separate locations on the shelves
- Reading back prescriptions, spelling out the name of medications, and providing the indication of the medication, when receiving a verbal prescription from the prescriber
- Emphasizing the use of methods such as "tall man lettering" to differentiate drug names

High-Alert/Risk Medications

High alert/risk medications refer to those medications that can cause significant harm to the patient when administered incorrectly or used in error. These medications generally have a narrow window of safety. Errors associated with high-risk medications result in devastating consequences to the patient and cause practitioners to suffer immense anxiety and guilt.

Here are some examples of high-alert medications:

- *Benzodiazepines*, primarily *midazolam*: used for sedation
- *Chemotherapeutic agents*: used for cancer treatment
- *Intravenous digoxin*: used to treat cardiac arrhythmia and heart failure
- *Dopamine, dobutamine*: used to treat depressed cardiac function
- *Heparin, warfarin*: used to prevent blood clots
- *Insulin:* used to control blood sugar
- *Lidocaine*: used to induce anesthesia
- *Opiate narcotics*: used for pain management
- *Neuromuscular blocking agents*: used as a muscle-relaxant or paralyzing agent
- Electrolyte solutions, e.g. intravenous sodium chloride, potassium chloride (or potassium phosphate), and magnesium sulphate

Pharmacies can use the following strategies to aid in avoiding errors associated with high-alert medications:

- Remove high concentration electrolytes from dispensing areas

- Use a leading "0" before the decimal place
- Avoid using risky abbreviations like "u" for unit or a tailing "0" on the dosage (e.g. 1.0 mg)
- Review LASA medications
- Use "tall man" letters for LASA medications
- Use colored warning labels
- Double-check dosage calculation independently

It is also necessary to pay attention to medications that should not be crushed as doing so could lead to high-risk situations. There are several reasons why certain medications should not be crushed:

- Dosage form is slow-release
- Dosage form is extended-release
- Dosage form is enteric-coated
- Mucous membrane could be irritated
- Possible increased rate of absorption
- Tablet coating could release the drug over a set period of time
- Taste
- Can irritate the skin
- Medication is liquid filled
- Dosage form is sublingual
- Dosage form is coated with a film
- Tablet is effervescent
- Potential for birth defects, teratogenic effect
- Acts as local anesthetic on the oral mucosa

A few examples of some medications that should not be crushed are *Cymbalta, Depakote, Prilosec,* and *Wellbutrin (SR, XL).*

Common Safety Strategies

A pharmacy should adopt and implement suitable strategies to prevent medication-dispensing errors. The following are some examples that can minimize medication-dispensing errors in a pharmacy.

Tall Man Lettering
Tall man lettering refers to the practice of using mixed case letters (uppercase and lowercase) to bring attention to the dissimilarities in LASA medication names. The Institute for Safe Medication Practices (ISMP) and the FDA encourage use of tall man lettering to decrease possible mix-ups of LASA medications.

Examples of Tall Man Lettering	
acetoZOLAMIDE	acetoHEXAMIDE
Chlorpromazine	chlorproPAMIDE
DAUNOrubicin	DOXOrubicin
Dimenhydrinate	diphenhydrAMINE
DOBUTamine	DOPamine

Separating Inventory

Dispensing errors can happen from mix-ups of the medications that are LASA or from medications that are packaged in similar ways. Mix-up errors can also happen from a medication with different strengths.

The following inventory management strategies can be implemented to minimize such errors:

- Label medications with both the brand name and generic name
- Use separate shelving for LASA medications
- Tag warning labels on high-alert medications
- Incorporate provisions in pharmacy software to alert users of LASA or high-alert medications

Understanding Leading and Trailing Zeros

A decimal point could be misplaced and lead to misinterpretation. The following strategies should be followed to avoid errors:

- *Leading zero*: A decimal point (a dose less than 1) should never be left "naked" and should carry a leading zero. It is often missed in fax prescriptions due to "fax noise." For example, without a leading zero, *.5 mg* of haloperidol could be misinterpreted as *5 mg* and cause overdosing.

- *Trailing zero*: A whole number should never be followed by a decimal point and a trailing zero. For example, with a trailing zero, *1.0 mg* warfarin could be misinterpreted as *10 mg* and cause ten-fold overdosing.

Limiting Use of Error-Prone Abbreviations

Some abbreviations could be misinterpreted and cause medication dispensing errors. It is recommended that pharmacies minimize the use of the following abbreviations in prescriptions, labels, and medication administration records:

Common Error-Prone Abbreviations			
Abbreviation	**Intended Meaning**	**Misinterpretation**	**Suggested Correction**
AD, AS, AU	Right ear, left ear, each ear	OD, OS, OU (right eye, left eye, each eye)	Use the written words instead (i.e., "right ear")
BT	Bedtime	BID (twice daily)	Use "bedtime"
cc	Cubic centimeters	"u" (units)	Use "mL"
IU	International unit	10 (ten) or IV	Use "unit"
IJ	Injection	IV (intravenous)	Use "injection"
o.d. or OD	Once daily	OD (right eye)	Use "daily"
qhs	Nightly at bedtime	qhr (every hour)	Use "nightly"
UD	"ut dictum" (as directed)	Unit dose	Use " as directed"

Practice Questions

1. Which information should be collected to ensure safe medication dispensing for a pediatric patient?
    I. Age and allergy
    II. Body weight
    III. Indication for the prescription
   a. I and II
   b. I and III
   c. II and III
   d. I, II, and III

2. You received a prescription of cephalexin for a 10-year-old child (body weight 66 lb.) suffering from impetigo. The direction on the prescription is "cephalexin 20 mg/kg/day QID for 10 days." Note that cephalexin suspension is on back-order, and the doctor's office is already closed. Thus, it's necessary to make a substitution. The pharmacist asks you to prepare the antibiotic suspension in sucrose syrup. How many cephalexin tablets (500 mg) are required to fill the prescription?
   a. 8 tablets
   b. 12 tablets
   c. 16 tablets
   d. 20 tablets

3. Which is NOT an effective strategy for preventing errors when receiving a verbal prescription?
   a. Collecting treatment indication
   b. Reading back prescription
   c. Spelling the drug's name
   d. Using abbreviations

4. To prevent a mix-up between chlorpromazine and chlorpropamide, all EXCEPT which of the following strategies will be applicable?
   a. Tall man lettering
   b. A computer alert for LASA medications
   c. Bar-code scanning of bottles at the filling station
   d. Better lighting on the shelves

5. Your pharmacy received an institutional order to supply 2 lbs of salicylic acid ointment (17% w/w) for treatment of warts. What is the quantity of salicylic acid required to prepare the ointment?
   a. 70.12 gm
   b. 80.32 gm
   c. 154.22 gm
   d. 170.78 gm

6. How many grams of 1% hydrocortisone cream should be mixed with an appropriate quantity of 2.5% hydrocortisone cream to make 250 grams of 1.5% hydrocortisone cream?
   a. 83.33 gm
   b. 166.66 gm
   c. 133.33 gm
   d. 116.66 gm

7. Who is the last person of defense to prevent a medication error?
    a. Physician
    b. Pharmacist
    c. Nurse
    d. Patient

8. Which of the following patient education strategies helps prevent medication errors?
    I. Encouraging the patient to review medications before leaving the pharmacy
    II. Educating the patient about medications dispensed
    III. Educating the patient about high-risk medications
    a. I only
    b. III only
    c. I and II
    d. I, II, and III

9. A physician called the pharmacy to give a verbal order of ZyPREXA 10 (olanzapine 10 mg). However, the order was misinterpreted, and the prescription was filled for ZyrTEC 10 (cetirizine 10 mg). Which of the following strategies would help to prevent such dispensing errors associated with LASA medications?
    I. The pharmacist reading back the prescription, including spelling the medication name
    II. The physician's office calling the patient and informing him/her that a prescription order has been placed at the pharmacy
    III. Counseling patient about the medication, including the purpose of the treatment
    a. I and II
    b. I and III
    c. II and III
    d. I, II, and III

10. You received a prescription of diclofenac (6% in diffusimax) gel for a patient with a sports injury. Given that the cost of diclofenac (250 gm container) is $95.00 and the cost of diffusimax (500 gm jar) is $85.00, how much would you charge the patient for a 100-gm gel? (Note that the professional/dispensing fee per prescription is $10.00, and the mixing fee is $0.02/gm/min. The average mixing time is 5 min.)
    a. $38.26
    b. $40.24
    c. $42.05
    d. $46.75

11. The strength of a medication in a prescription is written as 1%. The pharmacy technician feels that it might be too high of a dose, and it should probably be 0.1%. What should be an appropriate action for the technician to take?
    a. Ask the patient about the strength
    b. Fill the prescription as written
    c. Inform the pharmacist
    d. Call the physician's office to check the strength

12. Which of the following carries information about the pharmacology of a medication?
    I. Prescription label
    II. PPI
    III. Product monograph
   a. I only
   b. II only
   c. II and III
   d. I, II, and III

13. A patient brought a prescription for a medication with a direction of 50 mg tid for 10 days. The medication is available at a strength of 100 mg/5 mL. How many liters of solution should be supplied to the patient to complete the course of treatment?
   a. 75
   b. 95
   c. 0.075
   d. 0.085

14. To formulate 200 gm of an ointment mix from the ingredients A, B, and C with a ratio of 1:2:1, what quantity of each of those ingredients will be required?
   a. 40 gm, 120 gm, 40 gm, respectively
   b. 45 gm, 110 gm, 45 gm, respectively
   c. 50 gm, 100 gm, 50 gm, respectively
   d. 60 gm, 80 gm, 60 gm, respectively

15. Which of the following is the accepted convention for leading zeros?
   a. Use a leading zero with numbers greater than one (05 mg)
   b. Use a leading zero with numbers in decimal form less than one (e.g. 0.5 mg)
   c. Add a terminal zero (e.g. 5.0 mg)
   d. Increase the use of decimals, i.e. prescribe 0.5 g instead of 500 mg

Answer Explanations

1. D: All of the listed information is important. Confirming age and allergy are the primary requirements prior to prescription entry. Body weight is important because drug dose is based on weight. The indication of medication helps verify if the intention of the treatment matches with the prescribed medication.

2. B: The correct answer is *12 tablets*. Here's the calculation:

The body weight (in kg) of the child = (66 lb/2.205) = 30 kg (approx.)

- $Total\ child\ dose = Body\ weight\ (kg) \times \frac{dose}{day} \times number\ of\ days$

$$= 30\ kg \times \frac{20\ mg/kg}{day} \times 10\ days = 6000\ mg$$

Number of tablets required = Total dose/Tablet strength

= 6000 mg/500 mg

= *12 tablets*

3. D: Using abbreviations increases the chance of errors due to misinterpretation. For example, some abbreviations are particularly risky like writing "u" for unit or adding a tailing "0" on the dosage (e.g. 1.0 mg).

4. D: Better lighting will NOT prevent LASA medications mix-up as they are still next to each other on the shelf. Physical separation of LASA medications on the shelves, however, can reduce the possibility of mix-up.

5. C: The correct answer is *154.22 gm*. Here's the calculation:

Amount (in gm) of ointment = 2 lb. × 453.6 gm = 907.2 gm

Amount of salicylic acid required = amount of ointment × concentration of salicylic acid

= (907.2 gm × 0.17)

= 154.22 gm

6. B: The correct answer is *166.66 gm*. The calculation is below. Review the alligation method of pharmaceutical calculations.

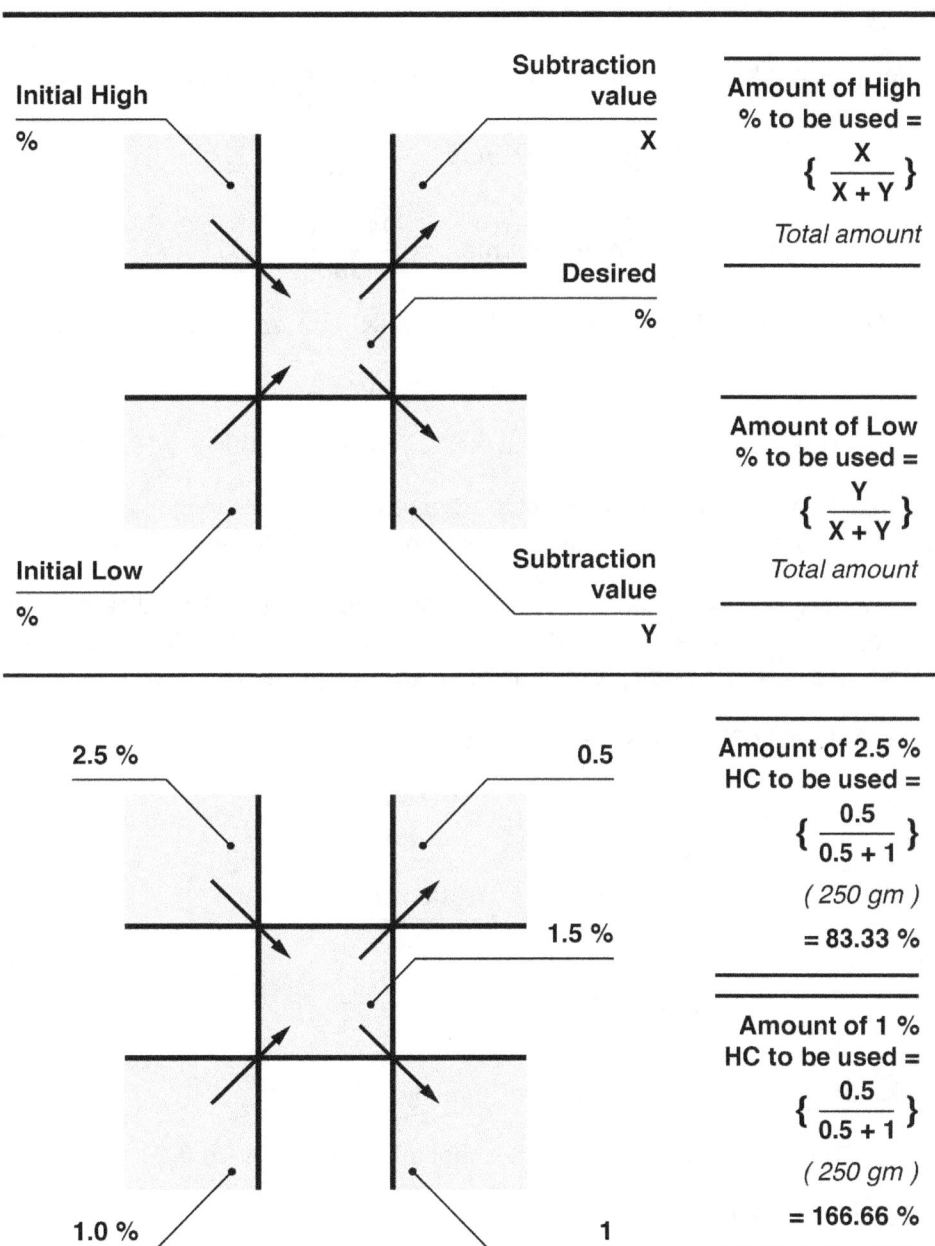

7. D: Patients are an integral part of the medication safety team. Patients should be educated about their medications and treatment objectives so that they can effectively contribute to preventing medication errors. It is recommended that pharmacists show medications to the patient at the time of dispensing, as this approach significantly decreases dispensing errors.

8. D: As mentioned, patients should be educated about their medications so that they can contribute to preventing medication errors.

9. B: Option II is incorrect because the physician's office did not inform the patient about the name of the medication and, thus, the patient cannot help prevent a medication error.

10. A: The correct answer is *$38.26*. Here's the calculation:

100 gm of diclofenac (6% in diffusimax) carries 6 gm of diclofenac and 94 gm of diffusimax.

$$i. Cost\ of\ 6\ gm\ diclofenac = \frac{6 \times 95}{250} = \$2.28$$

$$ii. Cost\ of\ 94\ gm\ diffusimax = \frac{94 \times 85}{500} = \$15.98$$

$$iii. Fee\ for\ mixing\ 100\ gm\ gel\ in\ 5\ min = .02 \times 100\ gm \times 5\ min = \$10.00$$

$$iv. Dispensing\ fee = \$10.00$$

$$Total\ charge = (i + ii + iii + iv) = (\$2.28 + \$15.98 + \$10.00 + \$10.00) = \$38.26$$

11. C: The correct answer is to *inform the pharmacist*. Choices *A* and *B* are inappropriate. Choice *D* is incorrect because communication with the physician is a pharmacist's responsibility.

12. C: The PPI (patient package insert) carries detailed information about the medication including the pharmacology. The product monograph or product insert (PI) or prescribing information (PI) carries various details of the medication including pharmacology, toxicology, and clinical studies.

13. C: The correct answer is *0.075*. Here's the calculation:

$$Total\ quantity\ required = 50\ mg \times 3\frac{times}{day} \times 10\ days = 1500\ mg$$

$$\frac{100\ mg}{5\ mL} = \frac{1500\ mg}{X\ mL}$$

$$X = \frac{1500\ mg \times 5\ mL}{100\ mg} = 75\ mL$$

As the question asks for the volume in *liters*, divide 75 ml by 1000:

The *volume* of solution to be supplied = (75/1000) = *0.075L*

14. C: The correct answer is *50 gm, 100 gm, 50 gm, respectively*. Here's the calculation:

Total parts of the ingredients (1:2:1) = 4

Quantity of A in 200 gm ointment mix = $\frac{1}{4} \times 200$ = *50 gm*

Quantity of B in 200 gm ointment mix = $\frac{2}{4} \times 200$ = *100 gm*

Quantity of C in 200 gm ointment mix = $\frac{1}{4} \times 200$ = *50 gm*

15. B: Using leading zeros with numbers in decimal form less than one (e.g. 0.5 mg) helps prevent dispensing larger doses for prescriptions. Choice *A* is incorrect because it does not make sense to include a leading zero with a whole number, and this option could be confusing to the reader. Choice *C* is incorrect because terminal zeros are not typically used as the decimal could be missed, and a ten-fold over-dose could be prescribed. Choice *D* is incorrect because the opposite practice is encouraged; that is, if it is possible to write a prescription without the use of decimal points, it should be done. Review section 4.6 for more details about leading and trailing zeros.

Pharmacy Quality Assurance

Any discussion of pharmacy quality assurance should begin with the differentiating quality control from quality assurance. *Quality control (QC)* refers to the process of routinely monitoring products to verify their suitability. The product or item being assessed by QC is typically recorded as correct or incorrect. QC assures the quality, purity, and efficacy of medications. It is governed by *standard operating procedures (SOPs)* and utilizes *good manufacturing practices (GMPs)*, which include daily control of quality, packaging, and storage conditions for medications. *Quality assurance (QA)* refers to activities implemented to assure the requirements for a product will be fulfilled without error. QA is also governed by SOPs and is tracked through audits. QA provides confidence on two fronts: first, internally to management; and second, externally to customers, regulatory bodies, government agencies, and any other third party.

There are many organizations that play a role in molding QA practices in the pharmacy setting. The *United States Pharmacopeia (USP)* establishes standards for the identity, strength, quality, and purity of medicines, food ingredients, and dietary supplements. The organization publishes the *United States Pharmacopeia and National Formulary (USP-NF)*, and all medications marketed in the United States must conform to USP-NF standards. Lastly, the USP-NF sets forth requirements for labeling of drugs, whether they are encountered in a multi-dose vial, unit-dose container, intravenous (IV) admixture, or compound.

The United States *Food and Drug Administration (FDA)* provides oversight for food, medicines, medical devices, blood, vaccines, veterinary products, biologics, cosmetics, tobacco, and radiation-emitting products. The FDA furnishes information on recent medication approvals, medication shortages, and drug safety information. The FDA also oversees clinical trials of drugs, submission of drug applications, and required labeling on medications. Finally, the FDA evaluates the safety of medicines, issues warning letters to the public regarding specific drugs, and conducts post-market surveillance of newly approved medications.

The Joint Commission (TJC) provides accreditation to various types of healthcare institutions including hospitals, nursing homes, physician offices, outpatient surgical hubs, psychiatric treatment centers, laboratory services, and long-term care facilities. Accreditation by TJC signifies an institution's dedication to the fulfillment of certain performance standards. The commission also provides certification for disease-specific care, advanced disease-specific care, palliative care, and home care. The commission also focuses on healthcare-associated infections, infection control, and patient safety issues, including medication errors.

The *Institute of Safe Medication Practices (ISMP)* provides impartial, timely, and accurate drug safety information. The ISMP provides pharmacy resources such as "do not crush" lists, black box warnings, error-prone abbreviations lists, confused drug names lists, high alert medications, and tall man letters. The ISMP also manages the *National Medication Errors Reporting Program (MERP)* and the *National Vaccine Errors Reporting Program (VERP)*. Currently, the ISMP is the only national nonprofit body concentrating on the prevention of medication errors.

Other organizations that influence pharmacy QA include the *American Pharmacy Association (APhA)*, the *American Society of Health-System Pharmacists*, the *Accrediting Council of Pharmacy Education*, state *boards of pharmacy (BOPs)*, the *National Association of Boards of Pharmacy (NABP)*, and the *Occupational Safety and Health Administration (OSHA)*.

Quality Assurance Practices: Medication and Inventory Control Systems

Inventory control may be utilized to provide pharmacy QA in a variety of fashions, including: ensuring that needed medications are available to provide treatment, establishing parameters for the proper dispensing of medications, removing expired and short-dated medications from inventory, regularly checking for drug recalls and performing all pertinent follow-ups, and separating inventory to diminish the potential for picking the wrong drug. Properly trained pharmacy staff, meticulous attention to detail, and automation are crucial for successful and dependable inventory control. Most pharmacies have established minimum and maximum inventory levels for the medications they stock. This practice ensures that an adequate, but not excessive, amount of a particular medication is stocked on the shelves.

Many pharmacies use computerized systems to monitor inventory levels. When a maximum level of a medication is reached, the pharmacy knows not to exceed that quantity and will hold off on reorders. When a minimum level of a medication is reached, the pharmacy will reorder. Controlling inventory levels helps with order fulfillment and minimizes the potential for drugs expiring while in inventory. Computer systems capable of tracking *National Drug Codes (NDCs)*, expiration dates, and lot numbers have added value and can help monitor for expired drugs, drug recalls, and can even interface with pharmacy management software.

Pharmacy personnel often are required to remove drugs from stock for reasons such as being expired, nearing their expiration date (short-dated), or being recalled. Proper inventory control and periodic manual checking of expiration dates helps to minimize the potential for dispensing expired medications. It also maximizes the usage of available stock before drugs become outdated. If an expiration date on a medication mentions only the month and year, the medication should be treated as expiring on the last day of the month. For example, a drug with an expiration date of 03/2019 should be treated as expiring on March 31, 2019.

Infection Control Procedures and Documentation

The goal of infection control is the prevention of healthcare-associated infections. These types of infections may be acquired in hospitals, outpatient clinics, rehabilitation facilities, nursing homes, or other clinical settings. The infections may spread from medical staff to patients, from patients to medical staff, from patient-to-patient, or among medical staff.

TJC mandates pharmacy infection control policies and procedures address the following:

- Hand washing technique and personal hygiene requirements
- Infection prevention, surveillance, and control
- Management and disposal of wastes
- Appropriate use of laminar flow hoods and monitoring them for microorganisms
- Preparation of irrigation solutions
- Preparation of sterile parenteral nutrition merchandise
- Periodic cleaning of facilities and the requirements for reporting unsanitary conditions
- Storage of sterile drug merchandise
- Periodic assessment of the use of sterile technique by pharmacy personnel
- Shelf-life of all sterile merchandise in storage
- Traffic control measures for sterile medicine preparation areas
- The use of single-dose and multi-dose containers

Measures implemented in the prevention of healthcare-associated infections include hand hygiene or washing and the use of *personal protective equipment (PPE)*. In the pharmacy setting, harmful microorganisms can be introduced into the laminar flow hood by coughing or sneezing without a mask in place, jewelry, loose facial and head hair, and cosmetics. As far as hand hygiene, the utilization of gloves does not waive the need for hand washing. Liquid soap is favored over bar soap. Hand washing is recommended in the following scenarios: before and after contact with a patient; after bathroom use; before eating, when hands are visibly dirty; and before donning gloves when working in the laminar flow hood. Alcohol-based hand sanitizers are sufficient if hands are not visibly soiled and traditional soap and water are unavailable. Hand sanitizer preparations should be applied to all hand and finger surfaces and allowed to air dry.

Items such as face masks, face shields, latex or nonlatex gloves, goggles, gowns, shoe covers, hair covers, and laboratory coats are considered PPE. They ensure a physical barrier is in place between medical personnel and specific substances such as drugs or blood. Face shields are recommended if splashes to the mouth, eyes, or nose may occur. Gloves should be changed every hour or immediately after soiling. Gloves should be removed in such a way as to avoid direct skin contact with the outside of the gloves. Employers must provide hypoallergenic, or nonlatex, gloves to staff with allergies to latex.

Medical personnel should know the proper sequence for putting on and removing PPE. For example, pharmacy staff must adhere to guidelines set forth in *USP 797*, a chapter on pharmaceutical sterile preparations in the USP National Formulary, when compounding sterile preparations. First, staff should remove all unnecessary outer garments and jewelry. Next, staff should put on shoe, facial, and hair covers, facemasks, and optional face shields. Then, staff should perform mandatory hand hygiene. USP 797 specifies:

"…personnel perform a thorough hand-cleansing procedure by removing debris from under fingernails using a nail cleaner under running warm water followed by vigorous hand and arm washing to the elbows for at least 30 seconds with either nonantimicrobial or antimicrobial soap and water."

After performing hand hygiene, staff should put on a gown with sleeves fitting snugly around the wrists. Upon advancing to the buffer area (a clean, sterile area), a waterless alcohol-based scrub should be carried out. Lastly, sterile gloves should be put on prior to compounding sterile preparations.

As more pharmacies provide injectable medications, there is growing concern over infections transmitted via sticks with contaminated needles. The practice of *needle recapping* affords reduced opportunities for accidental needle sticks. It is advisable to recap a needle on a syringe any time it is not used immediately. Needles should never be recapped using both hands and the needle should always be directed away from the body. A one-handed technique or a mechanical device designed to hold the needle sheath should be utilized when recapping a needle. The needles on disposable syringes should never be removed by hand. The practice of bending, breaking, or manipulating needles prior to placing them in sharps containers has been abandoned. Furthermore, advancements in medical engineering have provided safety needles and self-sheathing needles, which further reduce the risk of accidental needle sticks and sharps injuries.

Risk Management Guidelines and Regulations

Pharmacy personnel are responsible for providing dependable, safe, and effective care, which includes implementing strategies focused on the reduction of medication errors. *Risk management* refers to systems that identify, assess, and implement procedures aimed at reducing medication errors. Risk management has three components—QC, QA, and quality improvement. Pharmacies should include risk management guidelines and regulations in their SOPs. Risk management is an ongoing process and may require periodic adjustments.

Accuracy should be at the forefront of all prescription-filling activities. There are many medication error prevention strategies. Verification of patient information should be performed at every pharmacy visit. This practice is key in the reduction of allergic drug reactions and drug-drug interactions. There are various resources available on the Internet aimed at the prevention of medication errors. Pharmacies should also maintain an up-to-date library pertinent to the practice of pharmacy.

Advancements in pharmacy technology have made it possible to provide additional safety controls within the dispensing process. The order entry process can be automatically linked to the particular NDCs stocked on the pharmacy's shelves. As a result, the prescription label can be printed with a unique barcode linking it to a particular drug and patient profile. A barcode scanner can then be used to verify the correct medication is being used to fill an individual patient's prescription. In the hospital setting, barcodes can be incorporated into patient hospital bracelets, allowing hospital personnel to verify that the correct medication is being administered to the right patient at the correct time. The automation of pharmacy dispensing equipment has reduced medication errors.

The separation of a pharmacy's inventory by drug categories is another medication error prevention strategy. TJC mandates that external and internal medications are stored separately. The commission also requires separate storage of oncology medications and volatile or flammable substances. Oncology medications should be stored in a sealed protective outer bag to prevent potential leakage. Volatile or flammable substances should be stored in a cool environment with adequate ventilation. The storage area must be designed to minimize fire and explosive potential. Common look-alike and sound-alike medications should be stored in different areas of the pharmacy. Lastly, insulin brands should be stored separately from one another.

The prescription label should be compared with the original prescription by at least two pharmacy personnel. Electronic prescribing is favored over writing, telephoning, or faxing prescriptions to a pharmacy. Other medication error prevention strategies include questioning illegible handwriting, ambiguous orders, and uncommon or unfamiliar abbreviations. Prescriptions should utilize the metric system. Prescribers should always position a leading zero in decimal values less than one. Likewise, a trailing zero to the right of a decimal point should never be used. Mistakes with both leading and trailing zeroes may result in a dosage error of between a tenth-fold and ten-fold. It is advisable to double-count prescriptions of narcotics. Overall, a prescription order should be reviewed a minimum of three times by pharmacy personnel.

Medication error documentation may be accomplished with incident reports. Medication errors are numerous and varied, ranging from issues in filling the quantity or type of medication dispensed, errors reading a prescription or label, failing to verify a patient's medical conditions and any contraindications for a prescription, or dispensing a different patient's prescription to the wrong recipient. The individual staff member observing or initially informed of the incident should complete the incident report and turn it in to the supervisor on duty. Incident reports should contain the following information: specifics of the individuals involved in the incident (name, contact information, whether employee or patient), date, time, and location of incident, description of occurrence, type of injury, treatment provided (if applicable), name and signature of individual filing the report, and the date report was filed. The *MedWatch Program* is overseen by the FDA and provides an online voluntary reporting form. MedWatch also furnishes safety alerts for drugs, medical devices, biologics, cosmetics, and nutritional supplements. It is the FDA's "gateway for clinically important safety information and reporting serious problems with human medical products." The FDA also administers the *Adverse Event Reporting System (FAERS)* containing information on medication error reports and adverse events. The FDA also oversees the *Vaccine Adverse Reporting System (VAERS)*, which is a national vaccine safety surveillance database.

Communication Channels for Follow-Up and Problem Resolution

Communication channels are essential within the pharmacy, between professions (e.g., pharmacists or pharmacy technicians and physicians, nurses, physician assistants), between the pharmacy and third-party payers, and between the pharmacy and its customers to ensure excellent therapeutic outcomes. Within the pharmacy, personnel should be able to share information regarding drug recalls, drug shortages, drug back orders, and important patient-specific information. QA activities should focus on all of these areas to reduce medication errors and dissatisfaction among staff and patients. Pharmacy technicians routinely convey vital information to licensed pharmacists during the prescription-filling process. Important information can be disseminated in various ways, including emails, memorandums, bulletins and/or messages on white boards, and within pharmacy management software. *Channel richness* refers to the capacity of a channel to convey information effectively. The following list is assembled in terms of decreasing channel richness: face-to-face (most effective), telephone, email, written memorandums, letters, posted notices, and bulletins (least effective). The more information that can be exchanged during an encounter, the richer the channel of communication. Three characteristics determine the richness of a channel of communication. First is whether the channel of communication can convey multiple cues. For example, a face-to-face (most effective) exchange can convey verbal cues, tone of voice cues, and postural cues. Second is whether the channel allows for rapid bidirectional (both directions) feedback. For example, an email can be answered quicker than a written letter, which makes an email a richer form of communication than a written letter. Third is whether the channel of communication allows for personal focus during the exchange. For example, a telephone call is more personal than a posted notice.

Interprofessionally (between professions), pharmacy technicians and pharmacists often are required to contact physicians, nurses, third-party payers, and other medical personnel in their quest to provide quality healthcare. Reasons for communication may include obtaining approval for prescription refills or prior authorizations, clarifying of prescriptions, notifying potential drug-drug interactions, dealing with claim rejections from third-party payers, and verifying the information in a patient's profile. Many of these processes are automated, but some do require the clinical judgment of a licensed pharmacist.

Communication between pharmacy personnel and their patients is a critical task, because pharmacy personnel are responsible for both gathering and distributing information to patients. Pharmacy staff play a crucial role when a patient drops off or picks up a prescription: obtaining and verifying patient-specific information such as medical providers, medical diagnoses, drug allergies, and all current medications including prescription and *over-the-counter (OTC)* medications and dietary supplements. The collection of this data should be routine and ongoing at every pharmacy visit. The process ensures screening for drug-drug interactions and medication contraindications. Pharmacy staff can distribute information by providing counseling on medications (whether prescription, OTC, or dietary supplements), making medication guides available, and by ensuring all pertinent auxiliary labels are affixed to prescriptions.

An example of a situation requiring communication within the pharmacy, interprofessionally, and between a pharmacy and its patients is an FDA drug recall. Occasionally, drugs have to be recalled. Drug recalls can be initiated by the drug manufacturer, by FDA request, or by FDA order under statutory authority. Pharmacies may be notified of a drug recall either by mail or fax. There are three drug recall classifications—class I, class II, and class III. *Class I drug recalls* represent situations in which there is reasonable probability that the use of said drug will cause serious adverse health consequences or death. For example, the diet medication Fen-Phen® (fenfluramine/phentermine) was recalled due to reports of permanent heart valve damage and the development of pulmonary hypertension. *Class II drug recalls* represent situations in which the use of said drug might cause brief or reversible adverse health effects or where the chances of serious adverse health effects are remote. They are the most common type of drug recall. For example, injectable ketorolac was recalled due to the possibility of tiny particles in the vial. *Class III drug recalls* represent situations in which the use of said drug is not likely to cause adverse health effects. For example, fentanyl patches were recalled due to leakage of fentanyl gel, potentially exposing patients and their caregivers to the drug without applying the patch.

Occasionally, there are drug shortages, requiring notification of pharmacies, medical providers, third-party payers, and patients. Drug shortages may occur for various reasons, including manufacturing, supply issues, and the discontinuation of particular drugs by drug manufacturers. The FDA tries to minimize medication shortages and attempts to find alternative supplies of a particular medication from other drug manufacturers. Although drug manufacturers are not required to furnish specific information regarding drug shortages, many choose to do so out of respect for pharmacies, medical providers, third-party payers, and patients.

Productivity, Efficiency, and Customer Satisfaction

In the pharmacy setting, *productivity* refers to the number of prescriptions filled per pharmacist or pharmacy technician hour. *Efficiency* refers to the ratio of useful work performed by a pharmacist or pharmacy technician. Automation of pharmacies has increased both pharmacy productivity and efficiency with fewer medication errors. Automation to improve these processes may include barcode scanners, automated filling cabinets (e.g., ScriptPro or Omnicell®), and electronic pill counters. Furthermore, interfacing between automated processes and pharmacy management software systems can further streamline drug inventory control and improve a pharmacy's cash flow.

As a result of increased productivity and efficiency, pharmacies are realizing a real opportunity to increase *customer satisfaction*. Pharmacy customer service encompasses principles such as maintaining a positive attitude toward the customer; being friendly toward to the customer; not interrupting the customer; obtaining as much information as possible with each patient encounter; furnishing accurate information to the patient; understanding the customer's condition(s); preserving patient confidentiality; developing a professional relationship with each customer; demonstrating compassion toward the customer; supporting customer decisions; and avoiding conflict with the customer. Automation frees up pharmacists and pharmacy technicians to work on other tasks such as assisting with customers' questions, needs, and concerns. Customer service satisfaction may be measured in various ways such as surveys, follow-up surveys, and focus groups.

Practice Questions

1. Which of the following is NOT an organization that influences quality assurance (QA) in the pharmacy setting?
    a. United States Pharmacopeia (USP)
    b. Occupational Safety and Health Administration (OSHA)
    c. American Board of Internal Medicine (ABIM)
    d. American Pharmacy Association (APhA)

2. Which of the following organizations accredits and certifies more than 19,000 healthcare organizations in the United States?
    a. The Joint Commission (TJC)
    b. The Institute of Safe Medication Practices (ISMP)
    c. The United States Food and Drug Administration (FDA)
    d. The National Association of Boards of Pharmacy (NABP)

3. What is the correct time interval for pharmacy staff to perform mandatory hand hygiene prior to compounding sterile preparations?
    a. At least 10 seconds
    b. At least 30 seconds
    c. At least 60 seconds
    d. At least 90 seconds

4. What is the term referring to the number of prescriptions filled per pharmacist hour?
    a. Efficiency
    b. Quality control
    c. Quality assurance
    d. Productivity

5. What is the most common type of drug recall?
    a. Class I
    b. Class II
    c. Class III
    d. Class IV

6. As far as channel richness, which of the following is the most effective means of communication?
    a. Email
    b. Bulletins
    c. Letters
    d. Face-to-face

7. Which one of the following agencies may initiate a drug recall?
    a. United States Food and Drug Administration (FDA)
    b. Drug Enforcement Administration (DEA)
    c. Occupational Safety and Health Administration (OSHA))
    d. The Joint Commission (TJC)

8. Which of the following is the preferred method of transmission of prescriptions to a pharmacy?
   a. Writing
   b. Telephoning
   c. Faxing
   d. Electronic prescribing

9. Which of the following government organizations oversees the MedWatch Program?
   a. Drug Enforcement Administration (DEA)
   b. Occupational Safety and Health Administration (OSHA)
   c. United States Food and Drug Administration (FDA)
   d. The Joint Commission (TJC)

10. How should an expiration date of 03/2019 be treated?
    a. Expiring on March 1, 2019
    b. Expiring on March 15, 2019
    c. Expiring on March 31, 2019
    d. Expiring on March 24, 2019

11. Which of the following items is NOT considered personal protective equipment (PPE)?
    a. Underwear
    b. Facemasks
    c. Laboratory coats
    d. Gowns

12. Which of the following agencies oversees the National Medication Errors Reporting Program (MERP)?
    a. Drug Enforcement Administration (DEA)
    b. The Institute of Safe Medication Practices (ISMP)
    c. Occupational Safety and Health Administration (OSHA)
    d. The Joint Commission (TJC)

Answer Explanations

1. C: The ABIM is a nonprofit organization that certifies physicians who practice internal medicine and its subspecialties. Only physicians who demonstrate the knowledge, skills, and aptitude to engage in the health care of adults are certified. Choices *A*, *B*, and *C* are all organizations that play a role in molding QA practices in the pharmacy setting.

2. A: The TJC provides accreditation and certification services to more than 19,000 healthcare facilities in the United States, including hospital and non-hospital venues such as doctor's offices, nursing homes, home care programs, medication compounding facilities, palliative care programs, behavioral healthcare facilities, and laboratory services. The ISMP promotes medication error education and awareness, in addition to medication safety tools and resources. The FDA provides oversight for drug approvals and clearances, as well as drug recalls and alerts. The NABP is charged with protecting the health of the public.

3. B: USP 797 mandates that pharmacy staff remove debris from beneath fingernails using warm running water followed by brisk washing from hands to elbows with antibacterial or non-antibacterial soap for at least 30 seconds prior to compounding sterile preparations. Choices *A*, *C*, and *D* are incorrect as they all present the incorrect duration.

4. D: Productivity is a measure of the efficiency of production. In the pharmacy, it refers to the number of prescriptions filled per pharmacist hour. High productivity can lead to greater profits in business. Efficiency refers to the ability to produce a product or service without wasting time, energy, or materials. It is an important factor in determining productivity. Quality control (QC) seeks to maintain or improve product quality, while reducing or eliminating errors. Quality assurance (QA) refers to activities focused on ensuring a product meets certain specifications and customer satisfaction.

5. B: There are three categories for drug recalls. A class I drug recall is the most urgent type of recall as ingestion of the product being recalled may cause serious injury or death. A class II drug recall is the most common type of recall, and the drug being recalled has a remote probability of causing serious injury or temporary illness. A class III drug recall is the least serious of all recalls as the drug being recalled is unlikely to cause injury or illness.

6. D: Channel richness refers to the quantity of information that can be passed on effectively during an encounter. The more information that can be exchanged during an encounter, the richer the channel of communication. Three characteristics determine the richness of a channel of communication. First is whether the channel of communication can convey multiple cues. For example, a face-to-face (most effective) exchange can convey verbal cues, tone of voice cues, and postural cues. Second is whether the channel allows for rapid bidirectional (both directions) feedback. For example, email a richer form of communication than a written letter because an email can be received and answered quicker than a written letter. Third is whether the channel of communication allows for personal focus during the exchange. For example, a telephone call is more personal than a posted notice.

7. A: The FDA has the authority to initiate a drug recall, whether class I, II, or III. Reasons for drug recalls vary and may include health hazards, mislabeling, contamination, and manufacturing defects. In recent years, there has been a surge in drug recalls initiated by the FDA. The agencies in Choices *B*, *C*, and *D* do not have the authority to initiate a drug recall.

8. D: Electronic prescribing, or e-prescribing, allows physicians and other medical personnel to send prescriptions to a pharmacy electronically. This technology is quickly replacing other modes of prescription transmission such as written, faxed, or called-in prescriptions. E-prescribing has the advantage of providing the ability to transmit accurate, error free, and understandable prescriptions. As a result, it can decrease medication errors.

9. C: The FDA oversees the MedWatch Program, which is a safety information and adverse event reporting service (AERS). MedWatch focuses on drugs and medical devices. MedWatch is a voluntary reporting system and allows the information to be shared amongst healthcare professionals and the lay public. Reports are submitted via the Internet.

10. C: If an expiration date on a medication mentions only the month and year, it should be treated as expiring on the last day of the month. For example, an expiration date of 04/2019 should be treated as expiring on April 30, 2019. Since 1979, drug manufacturers have been required to print expiration dates on medications. It represents the last day a drug manufacturer can assure 100% efficacy and safety of a drug. The FDA establishes expiration dates for medications.

11. A: PPE is worn to decrease the risk of exposure to workplace hazards that may cause injury or illness. Employers are obligated to train and provide appropriate PPE to their employees. OSHA establishes the standards for PPE. Choices *B, C,* and *D* are examples of PPE.

12. B: The Institute of Safe Medication Practices (ISMP) oversees the MERP. The service provides for confidential and voluntary reporting of medication errors. The MERP performs analyses of the errors reported and circulates recommendations for their prevention to drug manufacturers and regulatory organizations. The ISMP also manages the National Vaccine Errors Reporting Program (VERP).

Medication Order Entry and Fill Process

Order Entry Process

<u>Pharmacy Technician Tasks</u>
During the order-entry and prescription-filling process, a pharmacy technician may be required to carry out a broad array of tasks, such as:

- Accepting new prescriptions
- Receiving prescription refills
- Asking prescribers for refill authorizations
- Gathering patient data
- Initiating and maintaining an electronic patient profile
- Entering pertinent information into the pharmacy management software system
- Interpreting prescriptions
- Billing prescriptions to third-party pharmacy benefit providers
- Counting and pouring medications
- Labeling prescription containers
- Returning medication stock to pharmacy shelves
- Repackaging medications
- Preparing unit dose medications

<u>Pharmacy Policies and Procedures</u>
Every pharmacy should have a standardized book outlining their particular policies and procedures, including a *mission statement* stating the goals and purpose of an organization. A book of policies and procedures is mandatory per regulatory and professional bodies (e.g., the American Pharmacists Association [APhA], the Joint Commission, and the American Society of Health System Pharmacists [ASHP]). Manuals for policies and procedures may be used as reference tools as well as for the promotion of workplace safety.

<u>Pharmacy Communication</u>
A pharmacy technician should be able to communicate with other pharmacy staff so work can be completed efficiently and safely. To that end, a pharmacy technician must have knowledge of common medical terminology and abbreviations.

Medical terminology is made up of *word parts*: roots, prefixes, and suffixes. These are combined to form medical words.

The following is a list of common word roots, prefixes, and suffixes (and their meanings) used in medical terminology:

Root	Meaning
cardi	heart
gastr	stomach
derm	skin
arthr	joint
pulmon	lung
hem	blood
gynec	woman, female
ped	child
ren	kidney
ophthalm	eye
rhin	nose
crani	skull
cyst	urinary bladder
encephal	brain
cephal	head
aden	gland
col	colon, large intestine
chondr	cartilage
cyt	cell
erythr	red
leuk	white
electr	electricity
onc	tumor
oste	bone
psych	mind

Prefix	Meaning
tachy-	fast
brady-	slow
uni-	one
bi-	two, both
tri-	three
hyper-	increased, above
hypo-	decreased, below
inter-	between
intra-	within
retro-	behind
dys-	bad, painful, difficult, abnormal
aut-	self
sub-	below, under
trans-	across, through

Suffix	Meaning
-logy	study of
-logist	specialist in the study of
-algia	pain
-it is	inflammation
-pathy	disease
-stomy	opening
-tomy	cutting into, incision
-ectomy	cutting out, removal, excision
-phasia	speech
-emia	blood condition
-phagia	eat
-uria	urine
-centesis	surgical puncture to remove fluid
-scope	instrument to visually examine
-scopy	visual examination
-megaly	enlargement
-oma	tumor, mass
-gram	record
-therapy	treatment

Pharmacy technicians may come across medical abbreviations and acronyms in prescriptions, medical charts, and varied forms of drug information. The following is a list of common medical abbreviations and acronyms, and their meanings:

Medical Abbreviation	Meaning
HIV	human immunodeficiency virus
AIDS	acquired immunodeficiency syndrome
BP	blood pressure
HTN	hypertension, high blood pressure
BM	bowel movement
DM	diabetes mellitus
FBS	fasting blood sugar
OA	Osteoarthritis
CAD	coronary artery disease
RA	rheumatoid arthritis
BPH	benign prostatic hyperplasia
CVA	cerebrovascular accident, stroke
DJD	degenerative joint disease
GI	Gastrointestinal
COPD	chronic obstructive pulmonary disease
CHF	congestive heart failure
GERD	gastroesophageal reflux disease
HR	heart rate
P	Pulse
NKDA	no known drug allergies
RBC	red blood cell
WBC	white blood cell
URI	upper respiratory infection
UTI	urinary tract infection
SOB	shortness of breath
ECG	Electrocardiogram
EEG	Electroencephalogram
IBS	irritable bowel syndrome
NPO	nothing by mouth
STI	sexually transmitted infection
PSA	prostate specific antigen
ANA	antinuclear antibody
NSAID	nonsteroidal anti-inflammatory drug
CNS	central nervous system
MS	multiple sclerosis
CXR	chest X-ray

Many of these abbreviations are derived from Latin and may be for routes of drug administration, dosage forms, weights, frequency of drug administration, volumes, names of drugs, and directions for compounding. Pharmacy abbreviations may be written in lower case or capital letters. They should be used with caution as misinterpretation can lead to medication error.

The following is a list of common pharmacy abbreviations and their meanings:

Pharmacy Abbreviation	Meaning
tab	tablet
cap	capsule
oint	ointment
g	gram
mg	milligram
mL	milliliter
mcg	microgram
U	units
NS	normal saline
PO	by mouth
IV	intravenous
BSA	body surface area
mEq	milliequivalent
IM	intramuscular
SQ, SC	subcutaneous
PRN	as needed
q	every, each
cc	cubic centimeter
gr	grain
ac	before meals
hs	bedtime
bid	twice a day
tid	three times a day
qid	four times a day
QS	quantity sufficient
QD	daily
QOD	every other day
0	hour
SL	sublingual (under the tongue)
au	both ears
ad	right ear
as	left ear
gtt	drops
ou	both eyes
os	left eye

od	right eye
amp	ampule
atc	around the clock
biw	twice a week
tiw	three times a week
wa	while awake
stat	immediately

Intake, Interpretation, and Data Entry

Prescription Intake

Per federal law, a pharmacy may receive a prescription order via one of the following methods:

- Written: The patient hands the original prescription to a pharmacy technician.
- Telephone: Also called a verbal order
- If the original prescription is for a non-scheduled II is a controlled substance, it may be telephoned in by prescribers or their representatives (e.g., a nurse).
- The patient may call in a refill for a prescription.
- E-prescription: Transmitted electronically
- Fax

It's becoming common practice for Medicaid, Medicare, and private insurers to track prescriptions using a prescription origin code (POC). The codes are usually entered into the pharmacy management software system and signify the following:

- 0 = Unknown (e.g., a transferred prescription)
- 1 = Written prescription
- 2 = Telephone prescription
- 3 = E-prescription
- 4 = Fax prescription

A prescription should include the following information:

- Date written: Prescriptions for non-controlled substances may be honored for up to one year after they are written.

- Prescriber information: Includes full name and title, office address, office telephone and fax number, and, if applicable, National Provider Identifier (NPI) number and medical registration/license number.

- Patient information: Includes full name and home address and, if applicable, weight, height, and allergies.

- Inscription: Includes name of medication, strength of medication, dosage form, and quantity to dispense.

- Subscription: Instructions to pharmacist.
- Number of refills
- Drug Enforcement Administration (DEA) number: Only required for prescriptions for controlled substances.
- Signature of prescriber

Prescription Interpretation

After intake, the pharmacy staff is obligated to understand and fill the patient's prescription. Prescription interpretation requires knowledge of the abbreviations mentioned above and may also require calculations to ensure that the proper quantity of medication is dispensed.

Prescription interpretation is ideal when the following elements are provided:

- Name, strength, dosage form, and quantity of medication to be dispensed
- Route of administration
- Frequency of administration
- Indication of whether a generic medication may be dispensed
- Number of refills: In the event the prescriber doesn't indicate the number of refills, it's assumed no refills will be permitted.
- If doubt exists when interpreting a particular prescription interpretation, a pharmacist should be asked to clarify.
- If the pharmacist cannot clarify, the prescriber should be contacted for clarification.

The following table illustrates some common dispensing errors:

Common Dispensing Errors

Prescriber's Intention	Misinterpretation
AD, AS, AU *right ear, left ear, each ear*	OD, OS, OU *right eye, left eye, each eye*
qod *every other day*	qd or qid *daily 4 times a day*
U or u *units*	Zero, causing a 10-fold increase in dose *eg. 4U to 40*
Trailing zero *1.0 mg*	1.0 mg mistaken as 10 mg
Naked decimal point *.5 mg*	.5 mg mistaken as 5 mg
Drug name and dose run together *Inderal40*	Mistaken as Inderal 140
Large dose without properly placed commas	100000 units mistaken as 10,000 units
AZT *zidovudine*	Mistaken as azathioprine or aztreonam

There are several types of prescription medication orders: STAT, ASAP, PRN, and standing. *STAT* refers to a medication order that must be filled within 15 minutes of receiving it in a hospital. *ASAP* refers to a medication order that doesn't have the priority of a STAT order, but needs to be processed as soon as possible. *PRN* refers to a medication order that may be filled or administered per patient request, but there are parameters set forth by the prescriber. *Standing* refers to a medication order that a patient receives at regularly scheduled intervals (e.g., one capsule every 6 hours).

Data Entry

After prescription intake and interpretation, *data entry* is the next step in the medication order entry and fill process. Information obtained by the pharmacy technician should be entered into the electronic patient profile. Most pharmacies use a pharmacy management software system for data entry. These systems are highly customizable, so no system may be the same as another.

Pharmacy management software may able to perform the following duties:

- Processing prescriptions
- E-prescribing
- Capability to capture signatures at prescription pick-up
- Providing a refill queue

- Managing workflow
- Scanning patient and prescription cards
- Verifying National Drug Codes
- Providing medication guides
- Adjudicating third-party insurance, including workers' compensation
- Processing of accounts receivable
- Performing POS (point of sale) transactions
- Online billing capability
- Managing inventory/stock control
- Automatic ordering of inventory through wholesalers
- Batch processing of long-term care (LTC) and nursing home orders
- Wireless capturing of signatures
- Electronic billing for medication therapy management (MTM)
- Providing support for compounding services

There are many of these systems competing on the open market, and they generally have one of two interface types: graphical use interfaces (GUI, pronounced "gooey"), and text-based interfaces. They all require the input of data.

Information in the electronic patient profile should be entered the first time a prescription is filled and picked up at the pharmacy. With each subsequent pharmacy visit, including new prescriptions and refills, the profile is updated, as it's crucial for the pharmacist to dispense the correct medication and decrease the risk for potential adverse effects.

The pharmacy technician follows prompts from the pharmacy management software to enter the correct information. Common information entered into pharmacy management software may include:

- Prescriber information
- Full name and title
- Office address
- Office telephone and fax numbers
- Medical registration/license number
- DEA number
- Patient information
- Name and home address
- Telephone contact (mobile, home, and/or work)
- Demographics, such as date of birth, age, gender, weight, height, and occupation
- Medical history
- List of current medications, including dosages and frequency of administration
- Medication/food allergies
- Payment type (insurance vs. cash)
- Relationship to cardholder (01 = cardholder, 02 = spouse, 03 = dependent)
- Third-party prescription insurance information
- Full name
- Coverage type (HMO vs. PPO) (primary vs. secondary)
- Bank identification number (BIN)
- Group number

- Member/ID number
- Prescription information
- Date written
- Patient information
- Subscription
- Inscription
- Signature
- Refills
- Prescription origin code (POC)
- Prescription number
- Dispense as written (DAW) codes, which insurance carriers use to determine a pharmacy's reimbursement and if the drug qualifies for complete or limited coverage. All pharmacies and insurance carriers use these codes. The DAW codes and their meanings are as follows:
- 0 = No drug preference indicated (generic substitution usually provided for cost savings)
- 1 = Brand-name to be furnished, and substitution not allowed
- 2 = Substitution allowed—patient-requested drug furnished
- 3 = Substitution allowed—pharmacist-selected drug furnished
- 4 = Substitution allowed—generic drug not available in stock
- 5 = Substitution allowed—brand-name drug furnished as generic
- 6 = Override
- 7 = Substitution not allowed—brand-name drug furnished as mandated per law
- 8 = Substitution allowed—generic drug not available in local market
- 9 = Other
- Drug information
- Drug name and (metric) quantity
- National Drug Code (NDC)
- Drug manufacturer
- Interactions/contraindications
- Auxiliary labels
- Lot numbers and expiration dates
- Stock availability
- Pricing
- Drug guides

Calculating Doses Required

Since physicians usually don't know how long a prescription will last, a pharmacy technician must be adept at an assortment of calculations. The first thing to master is the calculation of the days supply of medication, which indicates how long a prescription will last. It must be calculated not only for tablets and capsules, but also for injectables, liquid medications, inhalers, and nasal sprays, as well as for PRN (as needed) lotions, ointments, creams, and drops. Other tasks requiring calculations are adjusting refills and short-fills.

Days' Supply for Tablets, Capsules, and Liquid Medications
The most straightforward calculations for days supply are for tablets, capsules, and liquid medications.

Example: Calculate the days supply for a prescription written for penicillin VK 500 mg tablets #40 i tab PO q.i.d.

$$Days\ supply = \frac{Quantity\ Dispensed}{(Dose\ \times\ Frequency)}$$

$$Days\ supply = \frac{40\ tabs}{(1\ tab\ \times\ 4\ times\ per\ day)} = 10\ days$$

Example: Calculate the days supply for a prescription written for penicillin VK 500 mg/5 mL 200 mL i tsp PO q.i.d.

$$Days\ supply = \frac{200\ mL}{(5\ mL\ \times\ 4\ times\ per\ day)} = 10\ days$$

Calculations for PRN (as needed) tablets, capsules, and liquid medications are more complicated due to the variability of doses and their frequencies. In general, the calculation should be made using the highest dose with the shortest interval.

Example: Calculate the days supply for a prescription written for alprazolam (Xanax®) 0.5 mg #60 i-ii tabs PO q4-6h PRN anxiety.

$$Days\ supply = \frac{60\ tabs}{2\ tab\ \times \frac{24\ hours}{4\ hours}} = \frac{60\ tabs}{(2\ tab\ \times\ 6\ times\ per\ day)} = 5\ days$$

The results in the calculations above are even numbers. If the calculation yields a decimal, it's usually appropriate to drop the decimal.

Days Supply for Insulins
The majority of insulins contain 100 units per mL, and insulin vials are typically packaged as either 10 mL vials or boxes of 5 syringes containing 3 mL per syringe for a total of 15 mL per box. Insulin vials should be kept no longer than 30 days after being opened.

Example: Calculate the days supply for a prescription written for insulin glargine (Lantus®) 10 mL 40 units SC daily.

$$Days\ supply = \frac{10\ mL\ \times\ 100\ units}{(40\ units\ per\ day)} = 25\ days$$

Days Supply for Inhalers and Sprays
With inhalers and sprays, it's important to observe on the packaging how many metered inhalations or sprays are actually in a container.

Example: Calculate the days supply for a prescription written for a fluticasone (Flovent® HFA) 44 mcg inhaler ii puffs b.i.d. Each container is labeled as containing 200 metered inhalations.

$$Days\ supply = \frac{200\ puffs}{(2\ puffs\ \times\ 2\ times\ a\ day)} = 50\ days$$

Days Supply for Ointments and Creams
Calculations for ointments and creams are more complicated, because exactly how much is used per dose is unknown. Other complicating factors include the size of the area affected and the number of areas treated. In general, the directions are to use 1 gram (1000 mg) per dose per affected area.

Example: Calculate the days supply for Kenalog® cream 15g apply b.i.d to affected area(s).

$$Days\ supply = \frac{15\ g}{(1\ g\ \times\ 2\ times\ per\ day)} = 7.5\ days = 7\ days\ (after\ dropping\ the\ decimal)$$

Days Supply for Ophthalmic and Otic Medications
To determine the days supply for ophthalmic and otic medications, use a conversion factor to convert milliliters (mL) to drops (gtt). The agreed-upon factor is 20 gtt/mL. For ophthalmic ointments, a dose equals 100 mg.

Example: Calculate the days supply for pilocarpine 2% solution 15 mL ii gtt OU t.i.d.

$$Days\ supply = \frac{15\ mL\ \times\ \frac{20\ gtt}{mL}}{(4\ gtt\ \times\ 3\ doses\ per\ day)} = \frac{300\ gtt}{(12\ gtt\ per\ day)} = 25\ days$$

Example: Calculate the days supply for Neosporin® ophthalmic ointment 3.5 g apply OU q3-4h while awake.

$$Days\ supply = \frac{3.5\ g\ \times\ \frac{1000\ g}{mg}}{(200\ mg\ \times\ 5\ doses\ per\ day)} = 3.5\ days = 3\ days\ (after\ dropping\ the\ decimal)$$

The assumption, in this case, is that a patient sleeps 8 hours per day and is awake 16 hours per day. Using the shortest interval of dosing (every 3 hours while awake), the patient should apply approximately 5 doses per day.

Adjusting Refills and Short-Fills
Third-party prescription insurance providers often have dispensing limitations restricting the quantity of a medication that can be filled by a pharmacy. As a result, pharmacy technicians may have to adjust refills. The adjustment of refills oftentimes leads to short-filled prescriptions, or *short-fills*.

Example: A prescription is written for Celebrex® 100 mg caps #50 ℞ PO cap daily with 1 refill. The patient's insurance plan has a 30-day supply limitation. Calculate the number of refills and short-fills (if any) for the adjusted quantity.

First, calculate the total number of capsules over the life of the prescription:

$$50\ capsules \times 2\ total\ fills = 100\ capsules$$

Next, calculate how many capsules needed per fill:

$$Capsules\ per\ fill = \frac{1\ cap}{dose} \times \frac{1\ dose}{day} \times \frac{30\ days}{fill} = 30\ caps/fill$$

Next, calculate how many fills are needed to dispense the quantity as specified by the prescriber:

$$Fills = \frac{100\ caps}{(30\ caps/fill)} = 3.333\ fills$$

There will be at total of 2 refills after the initial fill by the pharmacy.

Now, calculate the quantity of the short-fill:

$$= \frac{100\ capsules}{3\ fills \times (30\ caps/fill)} = 10\ capsules$$

There will be a short-fill of 10 capsules.

Example: A prescription is written for Lexapro® 20mg #50 ℞ PO cap daily with 3 refills. The patient's insurance plan has a 32-day supply limitation. Calculate the number of refills and short-fills (if any) for the adjusted quantity.

First, calculate the total number of capsules over the life of the prescription:

$$50\ capsules \times 4\ total\ fills = 200\ capsules$$

Next, calculate how many capsules needed per fill:

$$Capsules\ per\ fill = \frac{1\ cap}{dose} \times \frac{1\ dose}{day} \times \frac{32\ days}{fill} = 32\ caps/fill$$

Next, calculate how many fills are needed to dispense the quantity as specified by the prescriber:

$$200\ caps/1 \times fill/32\ caps = 6.25\ fills$$

$$Fills = \frac{200\ caps}{(32\ caps/fill)} = 6.25\ fills$$

There will be a total of *5 refills* after the initial fill by the pharmacy.

Now, calculate the quantity of the short-fill:

$$= \frac{200\ capsules}{6\ fills \times (32\ caps/fill)} = 8\ capsules$$

There will be a short-fill of 8 capsules.

Caveat: Although pharmacy technicians are allowed to reduce the quantity dispensed in a fill, they cannot surpass the total prescribed quantity.

Fill Process

Once the order entry is complete, the next step is to fill the medication order. By this time, the pharmacy management software system has generated prescription container labels. The pharmacy technician must verify the information on the labels is accurate and error-free. The pharmacy technician pulls the prescribed medication from the pharmacy's stock only after verification of the prescription container labels. The medication on the prescription labels should be the same as the National Drug Code (NDC) number found on the bulk container. Scanning the Universal Product Code (UPC) on the bulk container should ensure the correct medication has been selected.

Next, the pharmacy technician must measure or count the prescribed medication. Counts are performed on a pill-counting tray. Counts can be made manually or with a machine. A recount of medication for accuracy is required, no matter the counting method. Manual counting should be done with a spatula in multiples of five.

After dispensing penicillin or sulfa medications, the counting tray should be cleaned by wiping it with 70% isopropyl alcohol. While dispensing oral chemotherapy or other hazardous agents, the pharmacy technician must wear gloves so the medication doesn't come into contact with the skin. In addition, the counting tray should be wiped with 70% isopropyl alcohol after dispensing the medication. Some pharmacies maintain separate pill-counting trays for penicillin, sulfa, and oral chemotherapy agents.

Next, the pharmacy technician should select an appropriately sized container and transfer the medication into the container. An appropriately sized child-resistant top should also be placed on the container. Patients are allowed to request an E-Z Open top. The pharmacy technician should ask the patient to sign the back of the original prescription to indicate that particular request.

The next step is placing the labels onto the medication container and upper-backhand corner of the original prescription. Currently, pre-printed auxiliary, or warning, labels should also be affixed to the medication container. The completed prescription container is placed on top of the original prescription with the bulk container that was pulled from the pharmacy's stock. The pharmacist checks and bags the prescription. The completed prescription is placed in the appropriate bin, and the bulk medication container is placed in its former position on the pharmacy's shelf.

Labeling Requirements

At a minimum, prescription container labels should contain the following information:

- Name, address, and telephone number of the pharmacy filling the prescription
- Prescription number (unique to the individual pharmacy)
- Manufacturer of the medication
- Date the prescription was filled or refilled
- Name of the medical professional prescribing the medication
- Patient's name
- Medication name, strength, and dosage form
- Directions for administration of the prescribed medication

- Quantity of medication to be dispensed (if a controlled substance, must be spelled out)
- Number of refills (if any)
- Initials of the licensed pharmacist dispensing the medication
- Expiration date of the prescription
- Any applicable auxiliary, or warning, labels

On prescription container labels for controlled substances, federal law mandates the following statement: "Caution: Federal law prohibits the transfer of this drug to any person other than the patient for whom it was prescribed."

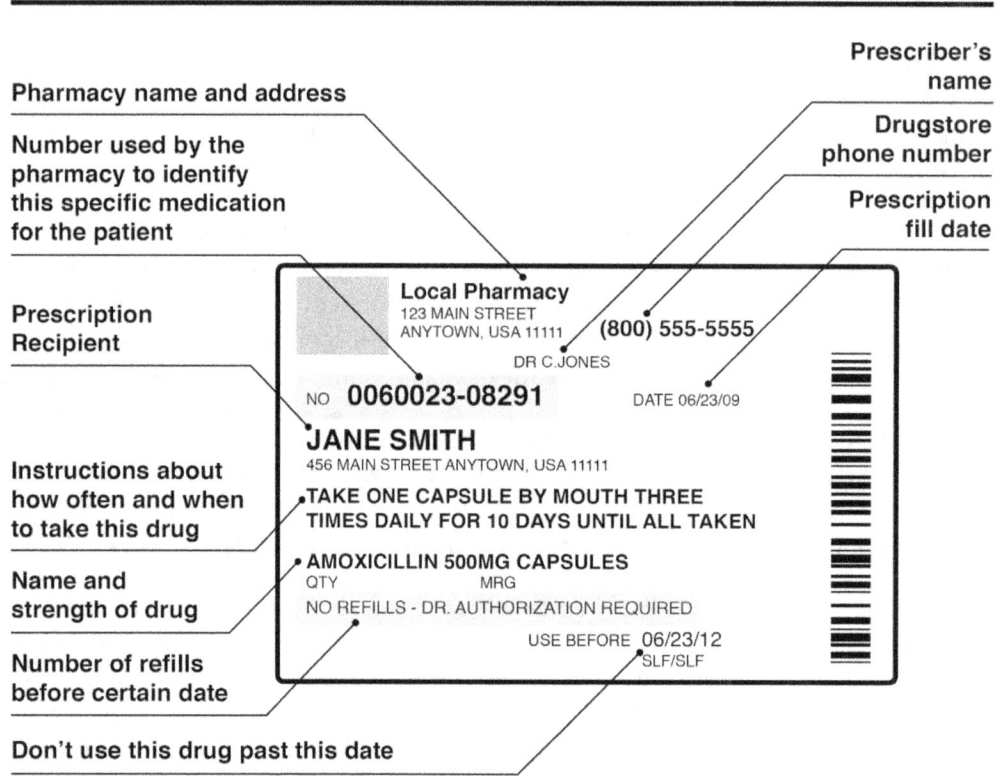

Auxiliary Labels
During the filling process, the pharmacy technician must affix any auxiliary, or warning, labels to the prescription container in addition to the standard pharmacy prescription labels. These labels are usually bright and colorful so they are noticeable. Auxiliary labels are intended to provide supplementary information regarding safe use, administration, and/or storage of the prescribed medication.

Common warning labels include:

- May cause drowsiness (usually recommended with benzodiazepines such as alprazolam [Xanax®] and antihistamines such as diphenhydramine [Benadryl®])

- Avoid alcohol (usually recommended with the antibiotic metronidazole [Flagyl®])

- Shake well (usually recommended with all suspension medications)
- Take with food or milk (usually recommended with nonsteroidal anti-inflammatory drugs [NSAIDs] such as ibuprofen [Advil®])
- For the eye (on ophthalmic drug preparations)
- For the ear (on otic drug preparations)
- For external use only or for topical use (on all ointments, creams, and lotions)
- For rectal use or vaginal use (on suppositories)
- Apply to skin (for patches)
- Avoid sunshine (for many acne medications)
- Do not crush or chew (for formulations of medications that are time-released)
- Take on an empty stomach (usually recommended with alendronate [Fosamax®] for the prevention and treatment of osteoporosis)
- Refrigerate (for some forms of insulin)
- Do not eat grapefruit or drink grapefruit juice (can increase blood levels of medications such as atorvastatin [Lipitor®], which is used to treat high cholesterol)
- Finish all this medication (important for medications such as antibiotics)
- Rinse mouth thoroughly after each use (usually recommended with inhaled steroids)
- Avoid wine, chocolate, and cheese (usually recommended for monoamine oxidase [MOA] inhibitors, a class of antidepressants)
- For the nose (on nasal preparations)
- Not for injection (medication should not be injected)
- Use as a gargle

<u>Medication Order Labels</u>
Other labeling requirements may be location (e.g., hospital vs. outpatient) or drug-specific.

The following are required on medication order labels (e.g., in the hospital):

- Name and location of the patient
- Generic or trade name of the medication
- Strength of the medication
- Quantity of drug to be dispensed
- Expiration date of medication
- Lot number of the medication

Sterile Product Labeling and Labeling for Repackaged Medications

Sterile product prescription labeling usually requires name of the pharmacy, patient name, date of filling, ingredients (strength and quantity of each), total volume, directions for use or administration, infusion rate, and beyond-use date. With regard to repackaged medications, only enough of the drug for a specified amount of time should be repackaged. Labels for repackaged medications require the name of the medication, name and address of the drug's manufacturer, strength and dosage form of the medication, beyond-use date, and lot number of the medication.

The repackaging log is required to contain the following information:

- Date that repackaging occurred
- Name of the medication
- Strength and dosage form of the medication
- Manufacturer of the medication
- Lot number of the medication
- Expiration date of the medication assigned by the manufacturer
- Beyond-use date (assigned by the pharmacy; cannot exceed the manufacturer's expiration date)
- Quantity repackaged
- Initials of pharmacy technician (if applicable)
- Initials of pharmacist

Unit Dose Labeling

The term *unit dose* refers to a medication used in the inpatient environment that's pre-dosed and pre-packaged from bulk into a single dose that can be administered to patients. The unit dose system made its debut in hospitals during the 1960s. Advantages of unit dose are ease of administration to patients, lower rates of medication errors (a barcode may be used for each unit dose), and reduced levels of medication waste. Disadvantages of unit dose are increased pharmacy processing time, increased cost of equipment, and the need for increased storage space.

Unit dose labeling should contain the following information:

- Generic or trade name of the medication
- Strength of the medication
- Name of the manufacturer
- Lot number
- Bar code (if applicable)
- Beyond-use date (assigned by the pharmacy; cannot exceed the manufacturer's expiration date)

Packaging Requirements

All medication leaving a pharmacy—whether inpatient or outpatient—must be packaged.

Ideally, medication packaging should be sufficient enough to:

- Protect against all adverse external environmental factors that could alter characteristics of a medication (e.g., light, moisture, temperature, and oxygen variables)

- Protect against physical/mechanical damage

- Protect against biological damage
- Provide identification and correct information for drugs

Types of raw materials used in medication packaging include cardboard, paper, glass, plastic, rubber, and metal (e.g., aluminum and stainless steel). The use of these raw materials generates a significant amount of waste. Methods of disposal of uncontaminated medication packaging include recycling, incineration (burning), and landfill. Cardboard, paper, glass, and metal are best disposed via recycling. Plastics and rubber are best disposed via incineration.

In general, packaging should maintain the stability of the medication while furnishing needed safety to patients and others who have to access the medication (e.g., caregivers and nurses).

Light Resistance
Medication packaging must have adequate light resistance. Currently, there are more than 200 medications that are sensitive to light. For example, when nitroprusside is exposed to direct sunlight, it changes into cyanide (a poison). The chemical composition of other medications may be altered by exposure to direct sunlight. As a result, many medications are dispensed in amber-colored containers. Common light-sensitive medications include doxycycline (Vibramycin®), linezolid (Zyvox®), acetazolamide (Diamox®), and zolmitriptan (Zomig®).

Child Resistance
In clinical trials, the implementation of child-resistant packaging has proven effective in reducing child mortality from oral prescription-drug intoxication. The three most common child-resistant closures are the "squeeze-turn," "push-turn," and a combination lock. Most medication containers considered child-resistant require two hands to open. This requirement may cause difficulty for elderly individuals.

The Poison Prevention Packaging Act (PPPA) of 1970 requires all prescription medications and controlled substances to be dispensed in vials with child-resistant caps. Exceptions to the legislation are few and may include a request by patient or physician not to receive the safety caps for oral contraceptives and select emergency sublingual (under the tongue) cardiovascular medications (e.g., nitroglycerin sublingually to treat angina associated with heart disease). If a patient or physician requests not to receive child-resistant caps, make sure that the back of the prescription is signed indicating the request for a non-child resistant container. The request should also be noted in the pharmacy management software system.

Medications dispensed or administered in inpatient environments (e.g., hospitals, long-term care facilities, and nursing homes) are also exempt from the child-resistant packaging legislation. A pharmacist's failure to abide by the PPPA could result in prosecution and imprisonment for no longer than one year, or payment of a fine of no more than $1,000, or both.

Storage Temperatures
Most medications may be stored safely at controlled room temperature. The United States Pharmacopeia has published the following standard parameters for medication storage:

- Freezer: Temperature maintained thermostatically between -13^0 and -14^0 Fahrenheit (-25^0 and -10^0 Celsius)

- Cold: Temperature not exceeding 46 ^{0}F (8 ^{0}C)

- Cool: Temperature between 46° and 59 °F (8° and 15 °C)

- Room temperature: Temperature prevailing in a working environment

- Controlled room temperature: Temperature maintained thermostatically between 68° and 77 °F (20° and 25 °C)

- Warm: Temperature between 86° and 104 °F (30° and 40 °C)

- Excessive heat: Temperature above 104 °F (40 °C)

- Protect from freezing: Freezing may lead to loss of potency or strength in a medication

- Dry place: Environment doesn't exceed 40% relative humidity

If the patient is to pick up medication from a community pharmacy, pharmacy staff should notify the patient of any special storage requirements. If the medication is being delivered by a pharmacy delivery service or mail-order pharmacy, special steps must be taken to ensure the medication is stored at appropriate temperatures (e.g., ice packs and coolers).

Containers and Container Materials
Medication packaging requires many different types of containers.

The following is a list of containers used in medication packaging:

- Round vials for capsules or tablets

- Wide-mouth bottles—for bulk powders or large quantities of capsules, tablets, and high-viscosity (thick) liquids

- Prescription bottles for low-viscosity (thin) liquids

- Applicator bottles to apply liquid medications to the skin

- Dropper bottles for otic, ophthalmic, nasal, or oral liquids requiring administration by dropper

- Hinged-lid or slide boxes for dispensing powders or suppositories

- Ointment jars and collapsible tubes to dispense semi-solid medications

For most medications, the original manufacturer's packaging suffices. In repackaging medications, pharmacy technicians should always be sure to consult the manufacturer's guidelines to determine if light-resistant packaging is required.

The following is a list of container classification:

- Tamper-evident packaging refers to a sealed container with medication intended for ophthalmic or otic use—a broken seal is evidence of tampering.

- A well-dosed container protects the medication from loss under normal conditions.

- A light-resistant container protects the medication from direct sunlight.

- A tight container prevents contamination by solids, liquids, or vapors.
- A hermetic container is unable to be penetrated by gas or air.
- A single-dose container refers to a single-unit container intended for parenteral (by mouth or the digestive tract) administration.
- A single-unit container holds one dose of medication.
- A unit-of-use container holds a specific quantity of medication that's ready to be dispensed but not yet labeled.
- A unit-dose container is a single-dose container for which the intended use is other than parenteral.
- A multiple-unit container allows for multiple withdrawals of a medication without affecting the quality, strength, or purity of the remainder.
- A multiple-dose container is a multiple-unit container intended for parenteral administration.

Other vehicles for the packaging of pharmaceuticals may include:

- Ampules: Single-dose containers sealed by fusion that can only be opened by breaking
- Bags: Containers composed of flexible surfaces with closed bottoms and sides that can be sealed
- Blisters: Multi-dose containers composed of two layers, with one layer constructed to hold single doses
- Bottles: Container with a neck and a flat bottom
- Cartridges: Containers to hold solid or liquid dosage forms (e.g., prefilled syringes)
- Gas cylinders: Containers capable of holding compressed, dissolved, or liquefied gas, and outfitted to regulate the flow of gas
- Injection needles: Hollow needles with locking hubs intended to administer liquid dosage forms
- Injection syringes: Syringes with or without fixed needles and freely movable pistons
- Pressurized containers: Containers capable of holding compressed, dissolved, or liquefied gas, and outfitted to produce the spontaneous, controlled release of a gas
- Strips: Multi-dose containers composed of two layers with perforations that holds single doses of solid or semi-solid dosage forms
- Tubes: Multi-dose containers made of collapsible material for release of semi-solid dosage forms released through a nozzle when package is squeezed
- Vials: Single- and multi-dose containers for parenteral medications containing an overseal and stopper

In May 1992, the United States Food and Drug Administration specified 11 technologies capable of fulfilling the definition of tamper-evident packaging. The list encompasses: blister and bubble packs; film wrappers; heat-shrunk wrappers or bands; bottles equipped with inner-mouth seals; plastic packs or paper foil; breakable cap-ring systems; sealed tubes; tape seals; plastic blind-end heat-sealed tubes; sealed cartons; all metal and composite cans; and aerosol containers.

A variety of plastics, including *polyvinyl chloride* (PVC), have been used in the last 50 years as materials for medication packaging. Plastics are an affordable option, keeping the majority of medications intact and uncontaminated. Plastics are unbreakable, light, and collapsible, which are significant advantages over glass. The main use of plastics is as material for bags for *parenteral solutions* (e.g., IV solutions).

Some medications may be able to bond with the PVC in containers, which may alter the structure and eventually harm the efficacy of a medication. In these scenarios, glass is a great alternative because it's *inert* (nonreactive). For example, sublingual nitroglycerin shouldn't be exposed at length to traditional PVC medication containers. Many pharmacists will dispense this medication in glass vials.

Metal is also used as a raw material in medication packaging. Metal is strong, impervious to gases, and shatterproof. Metal may be included in the structure of tubes, cans, blister packs, and pressurized containers (e.g., gas and aerosol cylinders). Aluminum and stainless steel are the predominant metals used in medication packaging.

<u>Syringes</u>
Pharmacies dispense two general types of syringes: oral/topical syringes and injectable syringes. Oral/topical syringes are perfect for precise dosing of oral or topical medications and have a safety feature that doesn't allow the attachment of needles. Injectable syringes are available in a wide assortment of sizes with numerous needle options. Historically, prescribers have been responsible for writing prescriptions for syringes and needles needed by patients. However, pharmacy staff may still have to determine the appropriate number of syringes and needles to dispense. In many states, patients are permitted to request syringes without prescriptions, although most insurance carriers don't cover syringes.

<u>Patient Package Inserts</u>
A patient package insert (PPI) is an informational leaflet written for patients that describes the potential benefits and adverse effects of medications. In other words, the PPI translates the technical language of the manufacturer's medication package insert into non-technical, or lay, terms.

The following information is required for a PPI:

- Description of the medication
- Clinical pharmacology (mode of action of a drug)
- Medical indications and usage
- Contraindications (reason to withhold or withdraw medication due to potential harm)
- Medication warnings
- Medication precautions
- Adverse reactions associated with medication
- Drug overdosing
- Dosage and administration of medication
- How the medication is supplied
- Date of the most recent revision of drug labeling

Pharmacists are required by law to provide a PPI to all patients receiving oral contraceptives, metered dose inhalers, menopausal products (e.g., estrogen, progesterone, and isotretinoin [Accutane®]).

Dispensing Process

Proper product validation uses National Drug Codes (NDCs), barcode scanning, and visual inspection/verification. The pharmacy technician should make a habit of checking the NDC in the pharmacy management software system against the product being dispensed. The practice not only decreases pharmacy error, but may also help avoid billing fraud. Many pharmacies use barcode scanning systems to provide another opportunity to reconcile the NDC in the computer with the one on the stock medication bottle containing the drug to be dispensed. Lastly, visual inspection is the oldest and most common form of verification. A registered pharmacist (RPh) traditionally carries out the validation, but some states allow pharmacy technicians to perform the task.

Visual inspection should verify the following:

- Accurate interpretation of the original prescription to the prescription label
- Accurate patient information on the product
- Appropriate packaging has been used
- Correct drug is being dispensed

After the medication has been filled and checked, it's ready for the patient to pick up. All new patients at a pharmacy should be given a copy of the Health Insurance Portability and Accountability Act of 1996 (HIPAA) notice of privacy practices. Pharmacy technicians must be sure to document the receipt of the notice by the patient. Per the Omnibus Budget Reconciliation Act of 1990 (OBRA-90), the pharmacist is required to offer medication counseling. The pharmacy technician may also feel compelled to offer medication counseling. If a patient would like to see the pharmacist for medication counseling, the request should be noted in the pharmacy management software system. The pharmacy should make a valid attempt at privacy for patient counseling sessions and may be achieved through a simple privacy screen or a dedicated room.

Pharmacy technicians routinely handle refills of prescription medication. Some refill situations require special attention, including:

- Early refill: Medication dosage may have changed or a patient may need a vacation fill. In some cases, insurance carriers have to be contacted.

- No refills: Generally, the prescriber must be contacted for a refill authorization. In some instances, the prescription may be greater than a year old, making it invalid.

- Controlled substances: Schedule II controlled substances cannot be refilled. Schedule III and IV controlled substances can only be refilled five times within a six-month period.

In 1970, the U.S. Food and Drug Administration (FDA) released drug classifications, or drug schedules, under the Controlled Substance Act (CSA). As mentioned, the drug schedules arrange drugs into groups based on risk of abuse or harm. Under the CSA, drugs and other substances considered controlled substances are divided into the following five schedules:

- Schedule I: These substances have no currently accepted medical use, a lack of accepted safety for use under medical supervision, and a high potential for abuse. Examples include heroin, marijuana, lysergic acid diethylamide (LSD), peyote, and 3,4-methylenedioxymethamphetamine (Ecstasy).

- Schedule II/IIN: Substances on this schedule have a high potential for abuse, which may lead to severe psychological or physical dependence. Examples include meperidine (Demerol®), hydromorphone (Dilaudid®), oxycodone (OxyContin®, Percocet®), methadone (Dolophine®), fentanyl (Duragesic®, Sublimaze®), morphine, opium, and codeine. Examples of Schedule IIN controlled substances include amphetamine (Adderall®, Dexedrine®), methylphenidate (Ritalin®), and methamphetamie (Desoxyn®).

- Schedule III/IIIN: These substances have less potential for abuse than substances in Schedules I or II, and abuse may lead to moderate or low physical dependence or high psychological dependence. Examples include combination medication products containing less than 15 mg of hydrocodone (Vicodin®) per dosage unit, products containing not more than 90 mg of codeine per dosage unit (Tylenol® with Codeine [Tylenol® #3]), and buprenorphine (Suboxone®). Examples of Schedule IIIN controlled substances include phendimetrazine, ketamine, benzphetamine (Didrex®), and anabolic steroids, such as testosterone.

- Schedule IV: Controlled substances on this schedule have a low potential for abuse relative to substances on Schedule III. Examples include carisoprodol (Soma®), clorazepate (Tranxene®), alprazolam (Xanax®), clonazepam (Klonopin®), midazolam (Versed®), lorazepam (Ativan®), diazepam (Valium®), triazolam (Halcion®), and temazepam (Restoril®).

- Schedule V: These substances have a low potential for abuse relative to substances on Schedule IV and consist primarily of preparations containing limited quantities of certain narcotics. Examples include cough preparations containing not more than 200 mg of codeine per 100 mL or per 100 g (Phenergan with Codeine, Robitussin® AC).

Pharmacies are increasingly using drug distribution systems that rely on automated dispensing systems. These systems serve as storage, dispensing, and charging (as in retail) hubs in a pharmacy. Automated dispensing systems simplify inventory control tracking, save time, and reduce medication errors. These systems are commonly implemented in hospital pharmacies and may be decentralized or centralized.

A decentralized pharmacy is housed in patient care areas, which is supposed to reduce or eliminate system management issues, such as poor recordkeeping and diversion of narcotics. Advantages of a decentralized pharmacy include the ability to document medication waste, dispense and return medications, and generate reports. A centralized pharmacy is used to improve the manual unit-dose cart fill process. The pharmacy technician usually hand-delivers medications to the unit in a centralized system. One disadvantage of a centralized pharmacy is the inability to stock all dosage forms of a medication.

Automated dispensing systems used in decentralized medication management include:

- Pyxis MedStation™ system: Barcode scanning ensures accurate dispensing of medications. Active alerts are also included to provide added safety precautions. It is considered one of the industry standards.

- Cubie™ system: Allows a nurse to access and remove only one medication at a time. The system reduces the risk of a nurse selecting a medication from the wrong pocket.

- Pyxis™ anesthesia system: Provides ease of access to medications needed by anesthesia practitioners by providing visibility to medication inventory. The system has biometric access and an array of drawer types.
- Pyxis™ CII Safe: Monitors and tracks the refilling of controlled substance inventory within a hospital.

Medication error is a leading cause of death in the United States. Dispensing errors account for 21% of all medication errors. Examples of dispensing errors include dispensing the incorrect drug, quantity, dose, labeling, or dosage form.

While previously discussed it is worth re-emphasizing strategies to minimize dispensing errors, including:

- Correctly enter the prescription: Transcription errors (such as omissions and inaccuracies) account for approximately 15% of dispensing errors. These errors may be reduced by consistently using reliable methods of verification while entering a prescription order into the computer.

- Confirm the prescription is accurate and complete: Pharmacy personnel should not second-guess ambiguous or illegible prescriptions. Other causes of medication error include the use of acronyms, nonstandard abbreviations, decimals, and call-in prescriptions. The prescriber should be contacted for clarification.

- Be aware of sound-alike and look-alike medications: Similar medication names account for 33% of medication errors. One example would be dispensing methadone instead of methylphenidate. Occasionally, these errors are fatal.

- Be careful with zeros and abbreviations: Misplaced decimal points or zeros and faulty units are frequent causes of medication error and are typically the result of misinterpretation. Misplacing a decimal point or zero may result in the patient receiving at least 10 times more medication than originally indicated. Stocking a single strength of a particular medication, computer alerts, and reviewing label instructions during patient medication counseling may reduce these errors.

- Keep workplace organized: In clinical trials, organization (e.g., work environment, workspace, and workflow) has been shown to markedly reduce medication dispensing errors. Examples of organization include adequate workspace and appropriate lighting. Pharmacy technicians should develop a routine for entering, filling, and checking pharmacy prescriptions.

- Reduce distraction: Distraction while working and multitasking are leading causes of dispensing errors. Automatic refill requests may reduce distractions. Factors that may influence work environments include window services, design of workflow, and automatic dispensing.

- Balance heavy workloads and reduce stress: Increased workloads have often been noted as contributing to dispensing errors. Sufficient staffing with appropriate workload assignments may help to reduce dispensing errors. These measures should also reduce stress, which may limit medication errors.

- Store drugs properly: Storing lookalike medications away from each other on the shelves can decrease dispensing errors. Always store stock medication with the container label facing forward. Locked storage for medications with a high potential for inducing errors is advisable.

- Thoroughly check all prescriptions: Checks and counterchecks of medication labels may reduce dispensing errors. For instance, check the written prescription against the NDC in the computer, the printed medication label, and the drug being filled/dispensed.

- Always provide medication counseling to patients: The vast majority of dispensing errors (83%) are identified during medication counseling sessions between the patient and pharmacist. These errors may be corrected before the patient leaves the pharmacy. Directions for use of medications should be covered during the counseling session, as misunderstood directions for use account for a significant portion of dispensing errors.

Practice Questions

1. What does the abbreviation PO mean?
    a. Daily
    b. By mouth
    c. As needed
    d. Bedtime

2. Which of the following pieces of information are included in the inscription?
    I. Medication name and strength
    II. Instructions for the pharmacist
    III. Quantity to dispense
    IV. Dosage form
    a. I, II, III
    b. I, III, IV
    c. I, II, IV
    d. All of the above

3. Which of the following statements is correct regarding ASAP and STAT prescription medication orders?
    a. ASAP orders, but not STAT orders, are only encountered in a hospital
    b. ASAP orders need to be filled within fifteen minutes of receiving them, whereas there is more leniency with STAT orders
    c. STAT orders need to be filled within fifteen minutes of receiving them, whereas there is more leniency with ASAP orders
    d. STAT orders, but not ASAP orders, are only encountered in a hospital

4. Calculate the days supply for a prescription written for alprazolam (Xanax®) 0.5 mg #120 1-2 tabs PO q4-6h PRN anxiety.
    a. Two and a half days
    b. Five days
    c. Ten days
    d. Twelve days

5. For how long can insulin vials be kept after they are opened?
    a. One day
    b. Seven days
    c. Thirty days
    d. Six months

6. Which of the following medications should be stored in glass rather than plastic?
    a. Doxycycline
    b. Sublingual nitroglycerin
    c. Linezolid
    d. Acetazolamide

7. Which of the following are advantages of decentralized pharmacies?
    I. The ability to document medication waste
    II. The ability to dispense and return medications
    III. The ability to generate reports
    IV. The ability to stock all dosage forms of a medication
    a. I, II, III
    b. I, II, IV
    c. I, III, IV
    d. All of the above

8. What method is most effective at reducing medication dispensing errors?
    a. Counseling sessions between the pharmacist and the patient
    b. Checking medication labels with the prescription
    c. Storing drugs properly and with labels facing forward
    d. Reducing distractions in the workplace and overworked staff

Answer Explanations

1. B: Pharmacy technicians should be familiar with prescription abbreviations. PO stands for per os, which means by mouth. Daily is QD, PRN is the abbreviation for *as needed*, and hs is the prescription abbreviation for bedtime.

2. B: The inscription should include the name of the medication, the strength and dosage form, and the quantity to dispense. The instructions for the pharmacist is part of the subscription. Both the inscription and subscription should be part of the prescription, along with information such as the number of refills, the prescriber's information and signature, and patient information.

3. C: There are several types of prescription medication orders. Both STAT and ASAP are relatively urgent orders that are received in hospital settings. STAT refers to a medication order that should be filled within fifteen minutes of its receipt. ASAP orders need to be processed as soon as possible but they are of lower priority than STAT orders. In contrast, PRN and standing orders are of much lower priority.

4. C: See calculation below:

$$Days\ supply = \frac{120\ tabs}{2\ tabs \times \frac{24\ hours}{4\ hours}} = 10\ days$$

Calculations for the days supply for PRN (as needed) medications are often more complicated than those with explicit dosage schedules due to the variability of doses and their frequencies. In general, calculations should be made using the highest dose with the shortest interval. In this case, that is two tablets every four hours.

5. C: Opened insulin vials should be kept no longer than thirty days.

6. B: According to the United States Food and Drug Administration's specifications for tamper-evident packaging, sublingual nitroglycerin should not be stored in plastic containers. The medication can bond with the PVC in plastic containers, which can alter the structure and eventually harm the efficacy of the medication. In those scenarios, glass is a great alternative because it is inert (nonreactive). Sublingual nitroglycerin is an example of a medication that should avoid prolonged exposure to traditional PVC medication containers. To combat this problem, many pharmacists will dispense the medication in glass vials because glass is inert. The other medications are light-sensitive, which means they should be dispensed in amber-colored containers, but they can be plastic.

7. A: Decentralized pharmacies are housed in patient care areas, in an attempt to reduce or eliminate system management issues such as poor recordkeeping and the diversion of narcotics by improving the manual unit-dose cart fill process. In contrast, the pharmacy technician usually hand delivers medications to the unit in a centralized system. Advantages include the ability to document medication waste, dispense and return medications, and generate reports. Unfortunately, such systems cannot typically stock all dosage forms of a medication, which is one downside.

8. A: While all of the options listed are important methods that should always be employed to reduce dispensing errors, counseling is the most effective method. The pharmacy staff should always provide medication counseling to patients. The vast majority of dispensing errors (approximately 83 percent) are identified in the counseling process. This important discussion between the pharmacist and the patient should be used to verify the medication, dosage and instructions for usage, and pertinent health information. Any errors or misunderstandings can be clarified and remedied prior to the patient leaving the pharmacy. Dispensing errors account for 21 percent of medication errors and can be fatal.

Pharmacy Inventory Management

Pharmacy Inventory Management

Although pharmacy inventory is simply defined as the types and quantities of drugs or medications on hand, pharmacy inventory management has a broader scope. With pharmacy inventory management, attention is given to procurement, drug storage and inventory control, distribution systems, and recollection and/or removal of consumed, unconsumed, and expired pharmaceutical products.

Pharmacy inventory management purposes are as follows:

- Help adequately furnish pharmaceuticals and pharmacy supplies
- Reduce stock-outs and temporary shortages that could affect patient care
- Reduce carrying costs of the financial investment in drug products
- Minimize the costs associated with placing orders to wholesalers
- Minimize the time spent on purchasing events
- Minimize inventory decline, breakage, and uselessness
- Decrease expenses by selecting products based on organizational formulary requirements, bioequivalence, and cost

There are different strategies for pharmaceutical ordering and inventory management:

Just-in-time ordering refers to ordering a medication prior to use. A pharmacy does not stock the item in its inventory; it is ordered only when a prescription is received for that medication. This strategy is useful for medications that are not fast moving, are costly, require special storage criteria, and are non-returnable. This ordering strategy helps to avoid holding up funds for an extended length of time, thus reducing inventory management costs and avoiding overstock and out-of-stock situations.

Automatic reordering, also called PAR Value or Periodic Automatic Replacement Value, is a system that alerts when a drug falls below a certain specified quantity. When considering product storage, space is of utmost important. Setting up the minimum and maximum for an item's inventory eradicates the guesswork when ordering medicine, as a predetermined number lays claim to the minimum and maximum amounts of drugs to be stored on the shelves. Historical data and current trends for an institution are considered to set up the minimum and maximum inventory of an item.

XYZ analysis is a method that identifies and defines items of inventory depending on their usage. The product is ranked based on its history of purchase and total annual costs. Products that have the highest inventory rate are prioritized, as shown below.

Rank of XYZ Item	Total Yearly % of Costs	% of Goods
X	80	20
Y	15	10
Z	5	70
Total	100	100

In the *80/20 rule*, 80% of a pharmacy's medicine costs result from 20% of the drugs carried. Therefore, attention is given to the inventory control of the medications in the top 20%. The inventory turn-over rate is the cost of items sold over the average inventory value. The goal is to make better use of the institution's financial resources by considering the integrating order costs and inventory holding costs.

In pharmacy inventory management, it is crucial to consider the types of inventories:

Types of Inventories			
Initial	**Biennial**	**Perpetual**	**Physical**
A precise inventory of all controlled substances accounted for before opening a new pharmacy or in the event there is a change of the in-charge pharmacist.	An inventory mandated by the Drug Enforcement Agency (DEA) of all controlled substances taken every two years. It requires a precise account for all Schedule II drugs, as well as Schedules III, IV, V, and "exempt narcotics" that may be estimated.	An inventory that requires exactly what is in stock at a particular time. Typically, perpetual inventories are upheld on Schedule II drugs, in addition to other drugs the pharmacy desires to watch.	An inventory performed mostly on a yearly basis. What needs to be determined is precisely what's in stock at a specific time and the value of the inventory based on the current cost of a drug at the time.

Function and Application of NDC, Lot Numbers, and Expiration Dates

NDC Number
The Drug Listing Act of 1972 implemented the National Drug Code or NDC as a 10-digit number, which distinguishes each and every medication used by humans. When one breaks down the 10-digit NDC number, each segment correlates specifically to the drug as follows:

- Labeler code is the first segment and refers to the manufacturer who produced the drug.
- Product code is the second segment and refers to the drug's strength and dosage form.
- Packaging code is the third segment and refers to the package size and type.

It is important to note that reassignment of an NDC number to a drug is prohibited, to avoid possible mix-up and to prevent health hazard to patients.

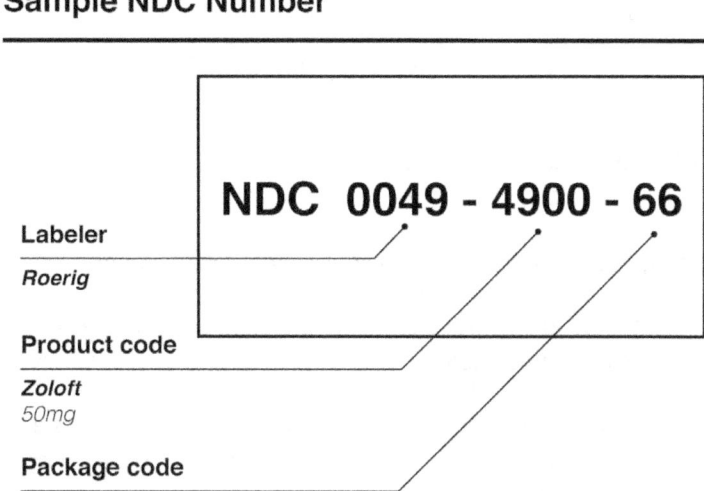

Sample NDC Number

Lot Numbers

To identify a product that has been manufactured, a lot number is assigned. A lot number helps track the product in the event of a recall. Lot numbers are usually assigned to a large batch of a product and placed on the retail packaging. This makes the product easier to track and trace back to its origin, even as it gets distributed nationwide.

Expiration Dates

For many pharmaceutical drugs, stability studies are performed to validate the potency, efficacy, and safety of a drug. Stability studies involve products placed in controlled experimental conditions, and followed by analytical laboratory testing to determine the expiration date of a drug. Some drugs are assigned a month or year expiration date, but drugs typically have a 12- to 60-month expiration date provided by the manufacturer.

Formulary or Approved/Preferred Product List

A formulary refers to the list of medications, as assigned by an institution/authority (e.g. hospitals, a particular health system, insurance, etc.), that are approved to be prescribed and/or dispensed. Following a formulary improves medication safety, efficacy, and cost-effectiveness. A formulary is maintained by physicians, nurse practitioners, and pharmacists. An *open formulary* is a list of all pharmaceutical products. A *closed (restricted) formulary* is a list of limited products in each drug classification; it limits the access of physicians to some medications.

Ordering and Receiving Processes

A number of terms are necessary to discuss in order to understand the ordering and receiving process of procurement. *Procurement*, which is defined as obtaining or buying goods and services, involves (1) drug selection, (2) source selection, (3) cost analysis, (4) group purchasing, (5) prime vendor relationships, (6) purchasing procedures, (7) record keeping and (8) receiving control.

These eight terms are explained in greater detail below:

- Drug selection involves cost analysis, including cost per dose, cost per day, or cost per treatment. It also includes a cost/benefit analysis, which investigates the cost of a drug versus the perceived benefits.

- Source selection simply analyzes if a drug – whether generic or brand name – should be purchased.

- Cost analysis involves analysis of costs associated with product acquisition, storage, associated fees, packaging, etc.

- Group purchasing organizations can purchase medications at lower costs relative to volume.

- Prime vendor relationships are established at the one source wholesaler, which supplies the majority of medications to a healthcare facility, institution, or pharmacy.

- Purchasing procedures involves coming to an agreement on discounts and settling payment schedules, terms of payment, prepayment policies, non-performance penalties, as well as policies for returned and damaged goods.

- Record keeping is most valuable, in that records must be managed to meet governmental regulations, standard of practice requirements, accreditation standards, polices, and management information.

- Receiving control—or more precisely, receiving procedures—involve shipments, invoices, and purchase orders that must be resolved by item.

Types of Inventory Ordering Process

Types of Inventory Ordering Processes				
Purchase from drug manufacturers	**Purchase from wholesalers**	**Just-in-time ordering**	**Point of sale**	**Purchase Order**
This process allows pharmacies to buy drugs in bulk, which creates savings for the company, because wholesalers may not have specific medications due to storage conditions, expense, or limited requests.	Since wholesalers stock drugs from all manufacturers, pharmacies may buy when they need a product rather than far in advance. Also, wholesalers offer additional services to pharmacies such as emergency deliveries and automated ordering systems or purchasing systems.	This method keeps inventory low and maximizes profit. The pharmacy can receive a drug the next business day after ordering, before running out of the product.	In the inventory system, a drug is deducted from inventory as it is dispensed. In many cases, the low inventory drug is automatically reordered.	To receive drugs and supplies from a wholesaler, a purchase order form must be completed. Information contained on the form can be found in the figure below.

A Sample Purchase Order Form

[Company Name]

[Street Address]
[City, ST ZIP]
Phone: (000) 000-0000
Fax: (000) 000-0000
Website

PURCHASE ORDER

DATE: 7/2/2017
PO#: [12345]

VENDOR

[Company Name]
[Contact or Department]
[Street Address]
[City, ST ZIP]
Phone: (000) 000-0000
Fax: (000) 000-0000
Website

SHIP TO

[Name]
[Company Name]
[Street Address]
[City, ST ZIP]
Phone: (000) 000-0000

REQUISITIONER	SHIP VIA	F.O.B.	SHIPPING TERMS

ITEM #	DESCRIPTION	QTY	UNIT PRICE	TOTAL
[12345678]	Product ABC	14	80.00	1,120.00
[87654321]	Product XYZ	10	25.00	250.00
[12341234]	Product MNO	1	50.00	50.00
				-
				-
				-
				-
				-
				-
				-
				-
				-

COMMENTS OR SPECIAL INSTRUCTIONS

Expected date of delivery

SUBTOTAL	1,420.00
TAX	-
SHIPPING	-
OTHER	-
TOTAL	$ 1,420.00

Receiving Processes
There are eight steps of the receiving processes:

- Verification of incoming items; i.e., drugs, dosage forms, strength, package size, number of units, and expiration date are matched against the packaging slip or invoice

- Personal protective equipment (PPE) must be worn by trained personnel when handling hazardous substances.

- Damaged or expired items should be recorded on the packing slip.

- Special storage items, such as items requiring refrigeration, should be promptly confirmed and put under required storage conditions to prevent spoilage, but more importantly, to prevent the loss of potency.

- The packing slip or invoice must be signed and dated.

- The required documentation is sent to accounts payable.

- When placing items on designated shelves, the drug with the oldest date should be arranged in front of those with newer dates.

- All applicable drug paperwork should be retained in the pharmacy as per the Controlled Substance Act, Occupational Safety and Health Administration, or the institution's policies and procedures manual.

Unit Dose Systems
Modern technology has allowed drugs or medications to be packaged in convenient and safe ways involving unit dose systems, which is when a medication is prepared in a labeled individual packet for convenience, safety, or monitoring. Unit dose packaging devices may be manual, semi-automatic, or automatic. The intent of a unit dose is to decrease administration error.

**A Unit Dose System:
A syringe as a final unit dose**

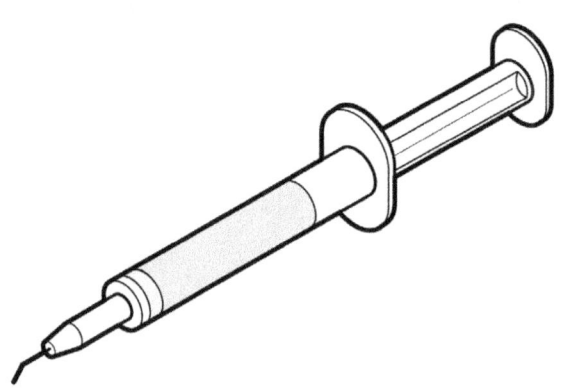

Modified Unit Dose System
A modified unit dose system is a drug delivery system that combines unit dose medications, which are blister packaged, into a multi-dose card instead of being placed loose in a box.

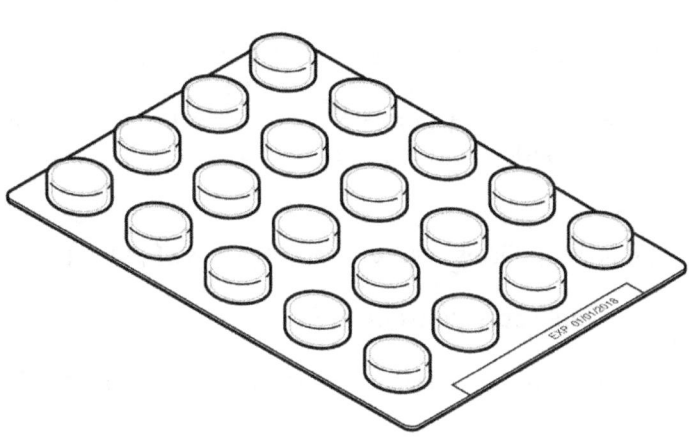

Pills in a Blister Pack

Blended Unit Dose System
A blended unit dose system is a combination of the unit dose system and non-unit dose system. It may contain multiple medications packed in a cassette. An example is a compliance (or bubble or blister) pack, in which multiple medications are arranged in each bubble (or compartment) according to the time of administration in a day or week.

Storage Requirements

Drug manufacturers determine specific storage conditions for the medications they produce. In addition, the drug manufacturer determines the type of container and temperature for storage of the medication. The temperature definitions have been defined in a previous section.

Removal

Medication Disposition
A drug recall can be opened by either the drug manufacturer or the Food and Drug Administration (FDA). The common causes for drug recall are serious adverse effects during post-marketing surveillance, formulation defects, formulation instability, lack of potency, packaging issues, delivery device (e.g. sprays or puffers) malfunctioning, and lack of good manufacturing practices. Poorly performed manufacturing practices involve a host of problems, such as unsanitary conditions for manufacturing a drug, which may constitute a recall.

Recalled Medication Processes
Six important steps are critical to the drug recall process.

- The manufacturer or wholesaler alerts the pharmacy/facility/institution via e-mail, mail, or fax about the reason for the recall. A recall notice contains the drug manufacturer's name, drug name, strength, package size, lot number or batch number, and expiration date.

- The pharmacy determines if the recalled medication is in stock. Physicians/clinics/institutions check if there are samples with that particular batch number in stock, and then contact the respective company representative for return of the samples.

- The pharmacy contacts patients who have taken the drug. Should the customer have the recalled drug, it must be returned to the pharmacy for a refund or substitute.

- The drug manufacturer directs the pharmacy to follow disposition directions.

- Drugs that have been recalled are returned to the manufacturer and returned for credit.

- The physician is notified of the recall and asked for a new order, especially if the drug will not be available for an extended period of time.

Expired Medications
- Each pharmacy establishes policies regarding the process of pulling drugs that will expire.

- Expired drugs must be kept separate from in-date drugs.

- Both pharmacists and pharmacy technicians must be familiar with the institution's policies regarding out-of-date drugs.

- Should a drug pass its expiration date before or during the course of treatment, it should never be dispensed to a patient. Depending on the contract with pharmacies and hospitals, wholesalers and manufacturers will determine if a drug will be returned for partial or full credit. Properly rotating drugs and employing sound inventory management skills can reduce the incidence of expired drugs.

- Cytotoxic drugs must be destroyed in accordance with the biohazardous waste management protocol.

- Reconstituted or compounded medication cannot be returned to the manufacturer. Partially used bottles of medication are often (but not always) non-returnable.

- Controlled substances with DEA numbers can only be returned by institutions. Long-term facilities cannot return controlled substances to pharmacies because they do not have DEA numbers.

- Destruction of controlled substances involves notifying the DEA at least two weeks before destruction. Form 41 is used for expired controlled substances and must be on file at the pharmacy for at least 2 years after destruction.

Pharmacy Waste

Pharmacy waste can be any chemically-manufactured good, vaccine, or allergenic used in the diagnosis, cure, mitigation, treatment, or prevention of disease or injury in humans or animals.

The following nine recommendations will minimize pharmacy waste:

- Make the best use of opened chemotherapy vials.
- Label medication for home use.
- Prime and flush intravenous lines with a saline (salt) solution.

- Check container sizes in relation to use.
- Substitute prepackaged unit dose liquids with specific oral syringes to patients.
- Get rid of stored controlled substances that are also hazardous waste.
- Use hard plastic buckets for delivering chemotherapeutic medication to hospitals.
- Monitor dates on emergency syringes.
- Review inventory control to minimize expired medications.

Pharmacy Waste Disposition

The following strategies pertain to waste disposal:

- Use hazardous waste labels to identify hazardous pharmacy waste.
- When not in use, keep containers covered.
- Limit quantity by allowing 3 days to dispose waste, once maximum capacity occurs.

Hazardous Waste

Characteristics of Hazardous Waste	
Ignitability	Flashpoint of less than 60°C.
Corrosivity	pH of less than 2 or greater than 12.5.
Reactivity	When in contact with water, this substance is liable to explode, react violently, or release toxic gases.
Toxicity	Toxic at a concentration above the limit of a regulated substance.
K-list waste	Contains one or more as corrosive, ignitable, reactive, or toxic substances.
P and U-list waste	Chemical matter that is commercially pure grade or technical grade, or a chemical formulation in which the chemical is the sole active ingredient.
Other	These substances are considered hazardous waste: • Medications with more than one active ingredient • All chemotherapy agents • Medications with low LD50s* • Endocrine disruptors • All drugs on the P and U lists

*LD50 (lethal dose) is the quantity of a consumed substance that kills 50 percent of a test sample. Its unit is expressed in mg/kg or milligrams of substance per kilogram of body weight.

Investigational New Drug

Drug manufacturers, institutions, or agencies will sponsor investigational drugs that are dispensed for a controlled study only.

The hospital pharmacy has the following duties:

- Distribution and control of investigational drugs, which involves drug procurement, storage, inventory management, packaging, labeling, distribution and disposition.

- Clinical services, which includes patient education, staff in-service training, and observing and reporting adverse medication reactions.

- Contributing to the preparation and review of research proposals and procedures, as well as helping with data collection and research.

Drug Approval Process

The drug approval process involves investigational drugs that are under clinical trials; however, they are not approved for sale in the United States.

There are 4 phases to the drug approval process: Phase I, Phase II, Phase III, and Phase IV.

- In Phase I, with regard to safety and toxicity, a determination of the appropriate range is made. Between 20 to 80 healthy individuals are selected for a 9- to 18-month clinical study.

- In Phase II, 100 to 300 subjects/patients who have the disease are selected for treatment. These patients are sometimes hospitalized for close surveillance. The focus is on the preliminary evaluation of efficacy and safety, where dose response and dosing schedule are paramount.

- In Phase III, several hundred to several thousand patients receive the investigational medication. It also involves a comparison between standard therapy or placebo and the investigational treatment. This phase may take two to five years to complete and it helps investigate the safety, effectiveness, and differences between the investigational drug and the control condition.

- In Phase IV, the post-marketing evaluation is conducted. It involves submitting an application called the New Drug Application (NDA) to the FDA for marketing approval. NDAs are submitted for approval after clinical studies are finished and the promoter believes that sufficient data exist to support the investigational drug's safety and effectiveness. Data are also collected from various treatment populations after the medication is marketed to evaluate the long-term safety and effectiveness of the treatment.

Ordering

The following constitute the necessary steps that physicians or researchers must perform in the process of studying investigational drugs:

- Researchers obtain approval from the Institutional Review Board (IRB).

- Researchers call the Interactive voice response system (IVRS) to initiate the screening and assignment of subjects for the study. A personal identification number (PIN) and password are given for tracing intentions. Physicians are provided with a facsimile (fax), which allows for drug supply reorder.

- Physicians complete the Investigational Drug Data Form and return it to the pharmacy.

- Doctors provide the pharmacy with a copy of the signed consent form.

- Doctors instruct manufacturers to give the pharmacy all pharmacologic and stability data.

- Physicians conduct arrangements for the transfer of the drug to the pharmacy.

- Doctors instruct the pharmacy to maintain a minimum level of the drug.

Receiving
The following steps should be followed when receiving a drug:

- A drug study must be accompanied with a drug shipment record.
- Upon arrival of the drug shipment, items must be recorded and stored appropriately.
- Shipment should match shipping records precisely.
- Any discrepancies in the type, quantity, lot numbers, and/or labeling mistakes with items in the shipment must be reported.
- The required quantity and lot number should be documented.

Storage
Investigational drugs must be secured in a location with limited access and a back-up power source. They should be separated from other drugs. Daily logs of storage temperatures and humidity should be maintained, with care that the identity, strength, quality, and purity of study drugs are not altered.

Accountability and Record
Keeping accurate drug records confirms that a drug study was distributed or applied according to the stated procedures. Dispensing records are stored for the sponsor of the study. Expiration dates and incremental dosing requirements should be reviewed and used to confirm the validity of study data and final outcomes. All records—from receipt to distribution to return—should be maintained for investigational drugs.

Investigational Drug Accountability Record
At the time of distribution of the study drug, the log book must be fully filled out with information about drug administration and signed. It should be re-checked; two people should initial the work. The Drug Accountability Record (DAR) must not have scratch-outs, white-outs, or any modifications. If an error does occur, a single line is drawn through the mistake, dated, and initialed and then the corrected information should be entered legibly at the time the event occurred. Backdating or pre-dating should not be used. All records must be orderly and clear and no extra line spaces can be included.

Patient Education
Patients should be instructed on how to appropriately use, handle, and return an investigational drug. They should be educated on the detrimental effects of missed doses, as well as not taking doses on time and any possible food or drug interactions. Patients should be advised that sharing of the study drug is prohibited. Bottles of the study drug must be returned.

Compliance
Compliance with a medication refers to a patient's adherence to the treatment and the directions of use of the medication. The common causes of medication non-compliance are unpleasant side-effects from the medication, lack of information/education, fear of use, and cost. The sponsor of an investigational drug should supply drug resolution education in written form. Once completed by the subject, it should be returned to the sponsor.

Pharmacy Security

Pharmacies are required to have a monitored alarm active when they are closed. In addition, pharmacies may install closed-circuit televisions. The safety of staff members, customers, and property are augmented when safety policies and protocols are in place. Pharmacies have the liberty to provide employee lockers in a safe area. In order to gain access to the pharmacy, a safe area to gain entry and sign for keys should be provided. Installation of motion detectors can provide added security during the off-hours. Pharmacy technicians are supervised by a licensed pharmacist, and only pharmacists or a designated employee should have access to close or open the pharmacy. Legal and institutional standards, as well as standards of practice, enforce access restriction to drugs with a sign "authorized personnel only." Employees should gain access to the specific area via touch pad and a scannable device for identification.

Financial Accounting Terminology

- Allowances: the seller gives the buyer a reduction in the buying price.

- Average cost method: a process to obtain the true per-item price by dividing the total cost to purchase a product by the number of units purchased.

- Consigned goods: items in possession of the consignee, while actual ownership of the items is in the hands of another party.

- Cost of goods available for sale: the price of items purchased and the totality of opening inventory.

- Cost of goods purchased: the sum of the net purchases and freight fees of all products.

- Costs of goods sold: the monetary difference in the value of opening inventory and ending inventory.

- Credit terms: the discounted price of items according to specific terms in a given time period.

- Current replacement cost: the current cost to replace an item in inventory.

- Days in inventory: the average number of days an item is held in inventory. It is calculated by dividing 365 by the rate of inventory turnover.

- Depreciation: the reduction in the tangible value of an item or business as its usefulness declines with time.

- First in, first out: the inventory process of selling the earliest acquired products first.

- FOB (Free On Board) destination: the items are the property of the seller while in transit to the buyer. Also, items are placed on board for free at the buyer's establishment, according to freight terms and the seller pays the freight fees.

- FOB shipping point: the items are the property of the buyer while in transit from the seller. Also, items are placed on board by the seller for the buyer according to freight terms, but the buyer pays the freight fees.

- Inventory turnover rate: the number of times inventory sold during a given time period.

- Last in, first out: the first items sold are the products that were most recently obtained.

- Lower of cost or market basis: used in certain accounting procedures when the value of the current product in inventory is less than it was purchased for so that its current replacement cost is less than its initial purchase price.

- Net purchases: the value of products available for resale after any purchase discounts or returns are subtracted from the total purchase price.

- Periodic inventory system: a system of inventory monitoring where items in stock are counted and compared with expected numbers based on purchases and sales over the same period.

- Purchase discount: a buyer receives a cash discount for prompt payment of a due balance.

- Purchase invoice: an itemized receipt of purchases provided to the customer from the seller.

- Specific identification method: items left in inventory are priced to get to the total price of ending inventory.

- Weighted average unit cost: the average price per item is found by dividing the total value of the items by the number of available products for sale.

Practice Questions

1. Which of the following terms pertain to Pharmacy Inventory Management?
   I. Procurement
   II. Inventory control and drug storage
   III. Label sensitivity and repackaging
   IV. Distribution systems and recollection
   V. Removal of consumed and unconsumed pharmaceutical products
   a. I, II, and V
   b. II, III, and IV
   c. I, II, III
   d. All of the above

2. Which of the following is NOT one of the seven Pharmacy Inventory Management purposes?
   a. Pharmaceuticals and pharmacy supplies are adequately furnished.
   b. Cost associated with placing orders to wholesalers is minimized.
   c. Inventory increase, breakage, and uselessness are minimized.
   d. Selecting products based on organizational formulary requirements, bioequivalence, and cost decreases expenses.

3. What process or method of pharmacy inventory management reduces inventory management costs and avoids overstock and out-of-stock situations?
   a. Economic order quantity
   b. Inventory turn-over rate
   c. Minimum and maximum
   d. Just-in-time ordering

4. Which of the following defines a perpetual inventory?
   a. An inventory mandated by the Drug Enforcement Agency (DEA) of all controlled substances taken every two years.
   b. An inventory that requires exactly what is in stock at a particular time.
   c. An inventory performed mostly on an annual basis.
   d. An inventory that is maintained automatically, based on order quantity received and prescription quantity dispensed.

5. There are three segments to the NDC number. Which segment identifies who manufactured a drug?
   a. Packaging code
   b. Product code
   c. Labeler code
   d. NDC code

6. Which of the following is true regarding lot numbers?
   a. They have the same digits as the expiration date
   b. They have a distinct number for each drug manufactured and supplied by the manufacturer
   c. They contain only numbers and no letters
   d. They can be used interchangeably among different drugs from the same manufacturer

7. Which of the following is not a valid type of formulary?
    a. Open
    b. Semi-closed
    c. Closed
    d. Restricted

8. Which of the following is NOT an ordering and receiving process?
    a. Drug selection
    b. Source selection
    c. Group purchasing
    d. Secondary vendor

9. Match the alphabetical letter of term with the corresponding definition.

Alphabetical Letter of Term	Definition
A. Point of sale	I. Pharmacies may buy when they need a product from a wholesaler rather than too far in advance.
B. Purchase from wholesalers	II. This process allows pharmacies to buy drugs in bulk.
C. Just-in-time ordering	III. In the inventory system, a drug is deducted from inventory as it is dispensed.
D. Purchase Order	IV. This must be completed o receive drugs and supplies from a wholesaler
E. Purchase from drug manufacturers	V. This method keeps an inventory low and maximizes profit.

   a. A = IV, B= III, C= II, D = I, E = V
   b. A = III, B = I, C = V, D = IV, E = II
   c. A = II, B = III, C = IV, D = V, E = I
   d. A =I, B = II, C = III, D = IV, E = V

10. PPE must be worn by trained personnel when handling hazardous substances. What does PPE stand for?
    a. Personnel provisional equipment
    b. Personal prescription evaluation
    c. Personal protective equipment
    d. Personal provided wear

11. Which of the following are not packaged in blister packs?
    a. Pills
    b. Topicals
    c. Encapsulated liquid pills
    d. Solid dosages

12. Who determines specific storage conditions and types of containers for manufactured drugs?
    a. Drug manufacturers
    b. FDA
    c. DEA
    d. Hospitals

13. In terms of severity and level of danger of a manufactured drug with defects, what is the order of reporting from greatest harm to least harm?
    a. Class II, Class III, and Class I
    b. Class I, Class II, and Class III
    c. Class III, Class II, and Class I
    d. Class IV, Class III, Class II, and Class I

14. How does the disposal of recalled drugs differ from that of expired drugs?
    a. It doesn't—they are both disposed of the same way.
    b. Recalled drugs require an investigation followed by destruction, according to guidelines from the manufacturer.
    c. Expired drugs require an investigation followed by destruction, according to guidelines from the manufacturer.
    d. Recalled drugs can be given to patients for 30 days after the recall has been initiated.

15. At the time of distributing and signing out the study drug, how many persons are responsible to re-check and initial the work?
    a. Three persons
    b. Only one person
    c. Two persons
    d. No person

Answer Explanations

1. D: All of the above terms pertain to pharmacy inventory management.

Procurement, drug storage and inventory control, repackaging and label sensitivity, distribution systems, and recollection and removal of consumed and unconsumed pharmaceutical products are all related to pharmacy inventory management.

2. C: The Pharmacy Inventory Management purposes listed do not include inventory increase, but breakage and uselessness are minimized; in contrast, inventory decline is minimized.

3. D: Just-in-time ordering is the strategy of ordering a drug just prior to use, which avoids holding up funds for an extended duration. This reduces inventory management costs and avoids overstock and out-of-stock situations.

4. B: A perpetual inventory is one that requires exactly what is in stock at a particular time. Usually, perpetual inventories are upheld on Schedule II drugs, in addition to other drugs the pharmacy wants to watch.

5. C: Labeler code is the first segment that reveals the manufacturer who produced the drug.

6. B: A lot number has a distinct number for each drug manufactured that is supplied by the manufacturer. It is important to note that drug manufacturers have their own system for numbering. A Lot number could, for example, be expressed as B11907. The B represents the initial of the company's name followed by in house numbering. Unlike an expiration date, it typically has the month and year expressed, for example as 06/2016, 06/16, or June 2016.

7. B: There is no semi-closed formulary.

8. D: Secondary vendor is not an ordering or receiving process.

9. B:

Alphabetical Letter of Term	Definition
B. Purchase from wholesalers	I. Pharmacies may buy when they need a product from a wholesaler rather than far in advance.
E. Purchase from drug manufacturers	II. This process allows pharmacies to buy drugs in bulk.
A. Point of sale	III. In the inventory system, a drug is deducted from inventory as it is dispensed.
D. Purchase Order	IV. This must be completed o receive drugs and supplies from a wholesaler
C. Just-in-time ordering	V. This method keeps an inventory low and maximizes profit.

10. C: PPE stands for Personal Protective Equipment. Personal protective equipment (PPE) must be worn by trained personnel when handling hazardous substances. PPE is a lab coat, rubber gloves, and safety glasses worn as a unit. PPE may include a breathing apparatus (mask) and/or outer jumpsuit made of protective material, in place a lab coat, when working in extreme hazard conditions.

11. B: There are various drugs packaged in blister packs from pills to encapsulated liquid pills (e.g. liquid Nyquil capsules) but topical ointments or medications do not come in blister packs. Only pills or solid dosages are packaged in blister packs.

12. A: Drug manufacturers determines the storage conditions, such as temperature, and other specifications for a medication.

13. B: Class I pertains to a reasonable probability that product use will cause or lead to serious adverse health events or even death, followed by Class II, which pertains to a likely probability that product use will cause adverse health events, which are temporary or medically reversible. Class III pertains to product use that will probably not cause an adverse health event.

14. B: Recalled drugs require an investigation followed by destruction according to guidelines from the manufacturer. Neither expired nor recalled drugs can be given to patients.

15. C: Two people should verify the work.

Pharmacy Billing and Reimbursement

Reimbursement Policies and Plans

Managed Care
This establishment offers healthcare and financing to their members with the goal of reducing unnecessary healthcare costs through a variety of mechanisms.

Managed Care Reimbursement
Managed care reimbursement involves capitation, which is a fixed, prepaid health service. The opposite is true for fee-for-service care, wherein a fixed fee is paid at the time that services are rendered.

Managed Care Providers
Health Maintenance Organizations (HMOs) strive to keep patients in good health. They aim for proactive healthcare as opposed to reactive healthcare. They survive on a fixed, prepaid services reimbursement structure. They predict payment costs for services. HMOs and healthcare providers work together directly.

Preferred Provider Organizations (PPOs)
PPOs offer discounted prices for members needing healthcare. They have non-exclusive contracts when working with providers. Copays are paid by members at the time of service. Yearly deductibles need to be met before a member's insurance coverage pays for services.

Point of Service (POS)
With a POS plan, members have the option to choose a HMO or PPO for healthcare. Medical care for these members are guided by the PCP. Members are allowed to choose out-of-network providers, but there are higher fees for out-of-network services, and premiums are higher as well.

Exclusive Point of Service (EPOS)
This service is a spin-off of a PPO, but this plan type does not pay providers who are outside the network.

Health Savings Accounts (HSA)
In order to pay for qualified medical expenses, a financial account called Health Savings Account can be set up. To take advantage of tax deductible contributions to HSAs, U.S. federal regulations mandate having a minimum deductible on health insurance for citizens. Both traditional and Roth 401Ks and IRAs, combined by HSAs for medical expenses, allow taxpayers to get a 100% income tax deduction annually on contributions.

Centers for Medicare & Medicaid Services (CMS)
CMS is a federal agency that is responsible for administering the Medicare program. CMS also works with state governments to administer Medicaid.

Private Plans
This type of plan is expensive to purchase. It is a prescription plan that enables the patient to receive benefits from a pharmacy.

Third Party Resolution

National Council for Prescription Drug Programs Rejection Codes
At least one rejection code will appear with a prescription claim that has been rejected. Before re-submitting the rejected claim to managed care, the pharmacy technician or pharmacist must fix the claim.

Rejection Description	Rejection Code
BIN (bank identification number), omitted or inacceptable	1
Version number, omitted or inacceptable	2
Transaction code, omitted or inacceptable	3
Processor control number, omitted or inacceptable	4
Pharmacy number, omitted or inacceptable	5
Group number, omitted or inacceptable	6
Card holder ID number, omitted or inacceptable	7
Person code, omitted or inacceptable	8
Birth date, omitted or inacceptable	9
Gender code, omitted or inacceptable	10
Patient relationship code, omitted or inacceptable	11
Date of service, omitted or inacceptable	15
Prescription/service reference number, omitted or inacceptable	16
Days supply, omitted or inacceptable	19
Compound code, omitted or inacceptable	20
Dispensed As Written (DAW)/product selection code, omitted or inacceptable	22
Prescriber ID, omitted or inacceptable	25
Unit of measure, omitted or inacceptable	26
Date prescription written, omitted or inacceptable	28
Number of refills authorized, omitted or inacceptable	29

Prior Authorization
Processing the prescription for certain medications requires the prescribing physician to get an approval from a managed care establishment. This process is called *prior authorization*. Prior authorization is an added step in the prescription billing process, and must take place before the insurance company will pay for the prescription. Therefore, if a prescription has not been approved by the insurance company, the patient may be responsible for the entire cost.

Conditions that may require prior authorization for a prescription include:

- Generic medications available but the brand name is specifically requested
- Expensive medications
- Drugs with age restrictions or limits
- Cosmetic drugs
- Non-life threatening drug use purposes only
- Necessary for treatment according to the physician, but not covered by the insurance
- Higher than normal dose

Third-Party Reimbursement Systems

Pharmacy Benefit Manager (PMB)
PMB is a third party that operates prescription drug programs for various agencies or institutions, including Medicare Part D plans, federal and state government employee benefits programs, commercial health plans, and self-insured employer plans. They are responsible for developing and maintaining formularies; negotiating prices, discounts, and rebates with manufacturers; and processing and paying prescription claims.

Medication Assistance Programs
Qualified patients, who are not able to pay for their medications, may participate in the medication assistance program, formed by drug manufacturers and other organizations. In this process, the patient mails an application and financial information. The physician needs to provide information about the prescription. The manufacturer reviews the application and informs the patient if he or she is eligible to receives assistance. Medication assistance programs are also provided by states and by non-profit groups; however, the requirements for eligibility might vary.

Coupons
Manufacturers sometimes create coupons for certain medications, especially if they are new drugs. Physicians give these coupons to patients upon receiving a new prescription. For the value of the coupon, the drug manufacturer is sent a bill electronically from the pharmacy.

Self-Pay
When the patient is required to pay the entire fee or full price of a prescription, the patient may pay by cash, check, credit, or debit card.

Healthcare Reimbursement Systems

Home Health, Long-Term Care, and Home Infusion
Home healthcare helps a patient receive treatment independently at home, which can delay the need to move to a long-term care facility. Home health program may include short-term and long-term care, dialysis, intravenous therapy, nursing, counseling, physiotherapy, etc. Home infusion programs include administration of intravenous medications, including antibiotics and chemotherapy, at the patient's own home.

Pharmacy Reimbursement from Managed Care
The formulas below detail the pharmacy reimbursement from managed care:

$$\text{Reimbursement Formula} = \text{Ingredient cost} + \text{Dispensing fee}$$

Dispensing fees are expressed as a dollar amount that is predetermined or a dollar amount as a percentage.

The average wholesale price (AWP) is the average price of medicine sold by wholesalers, expressed as:

Managed Care Reimbursement Formula = AWP − % Discount + Dispensing fee

Note that discounts based on volume are not considered. AWP is not a government-regulated price.

Actual Acquisition Cost (AAC) Formula = AAC + Dispensing fee

The Actual Acquisition Cost represents the price that the pharmacy actually paid to obtain a medicine.

Maximum Allowable Cost (MAC), expressed as MAC + Dispensing fee, is the reimbursement formula for generic medicines. Managed care oversees the outcome of MAC.

Formulary Usage in Managed Care
Under a prescription plan, there is a list of drugs approved for consumption or reimbursement. Each managed care establishment decides for themselves which formulary to use to control the cost of prescriptions.

Four major formularies exist:

- Open formulary: This list contains a selection of many medicines in each medicinal group. Multiple tiers of pricing exist and there is different pricing for generic medications, brand name medications, lifestyle medications, and medications not covered on the formulary.

- Closed formulary: This list contains just a few medicines for each therapeutic group. In some cases, a whole group of medicines is not accessible.

- Restricted formulary: This list contains a partly closed list, which is limited and selective.

- Formulary exception process: This list contains selected non-formulary and formulary drugs to be dispersed. The process may involve a formulary override, a process by which a doctor, upon approval, prescribes a non-formulary drug. In this process, prior authorization is obtained to use non-formulary medicines, which require the doctor to request the drug, and document the reason why the drug is medically necessary.

Online Adjudication
When filling a prescription, to guarantee precise copayments and timely payments, a pharmacy submits an electronic prescription claim to a third party provider.

Prescription Processing

Information contained on a prescription card can be seen below.

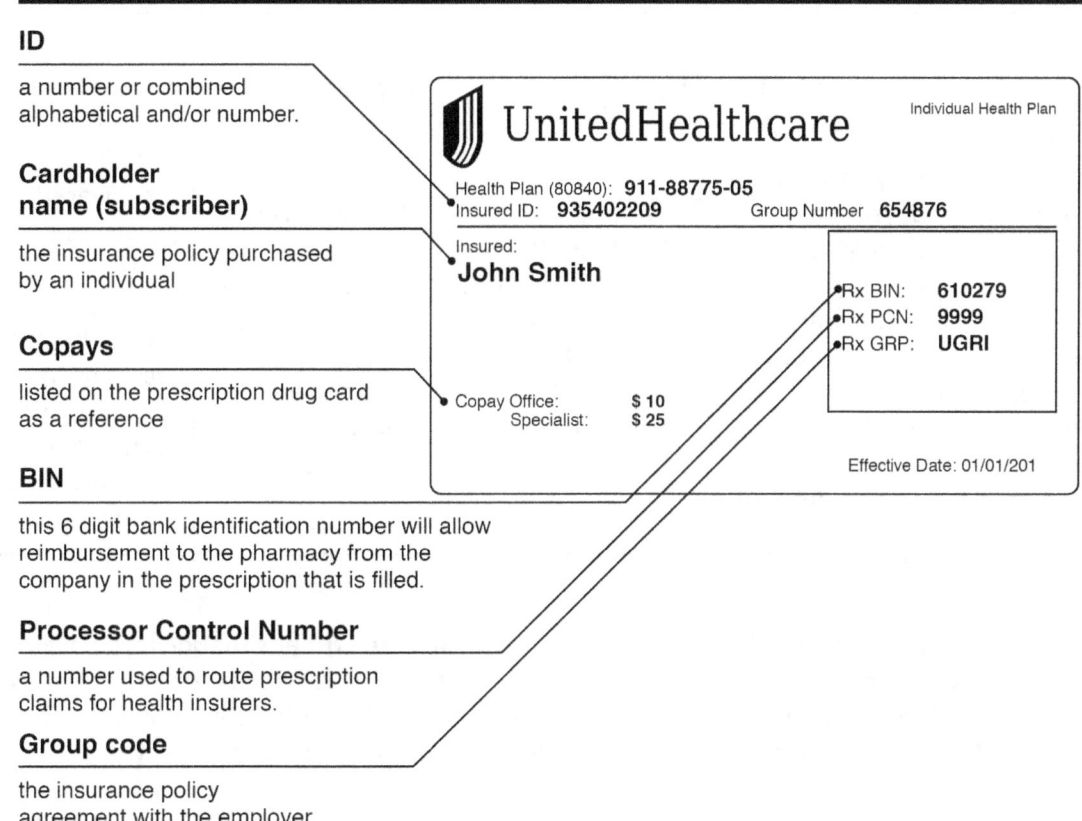

The nine DAW codes, previously mentioned, are listed again below:

Dispense As Written (DAW) Codes	Number
There is no indication of product selection.	0
Provider does not allow substitution.	1
When a patient requesting a drug to be dispensed, substitution is allowed.	2
When a pharmacist selecting a drug to be dispensed, substitution is allowed.	3
When generic drugs are not in stock, substitution is allowed.	4
When a brand name drug is dispensed as a generic drug, substitution is allowed.	5
Supersede.	6
When a brand name drug is mandated by law, substitution is not allowed.	7
When a generic drug is not available, substitution is allowed.	8
Additional.	9

Coordination of Benefits

Federally Funded Healthcare Programs: Medicare and Medicaid

Medicare is a federal program to provide healthcare for the elderly, disabled, and end stage kidney disease patients. The program includes Medicare Part A, Medicare Part B, Medicare Advantage (Part C), Medigap (Medicare Supplement Policy), and Medicare Part D.

Medicare Plans				
Medicare Part A	Medicare Part B	Medicare Advantage	Medigap	Medicare Part D
Insures home healthcare, hospice (palliative care), nursing homes, and inpatient hospital care. If the subscriber worked 10 years for a Medicare-provided employer, there is no fee.	Insures some physical and occupational therapy, outpatient care, and services by the physician. Additional monthly payments are required.	Partakers in Medicare Part A and B are allowed to get coverage via HMO or PPO for added services at a higher premium.	Participants can purchase an additional policy to cover gaps in medical expenses not covered by Medicare.	Not all medicines are covered under Medicare Part D; however, prescription drugs and biologicals, including insulin, vaccines, and certain medical supplies, are covered.

Medicaid

Participation in the federal Medicaid program is based on income and other situations. The eligibility rules, provided services, and co-pays are determined by each state, but eligibility for benefits is usually evaluated on a month-to-month basis. Depending on the circumstances, Medicaid provides coverage for doctor's appointments, emergency visits, hospitals, vaccines, and children's preventative care.

Pharmacy Provider Networks

Definitions and descriptions for pharmacy provider networks are listed below:

- Network: Providing healthcare services to members in a network of provider connected by a contract.

- Community Pharmacy Network: Combined as independent and pharmacy chains that may be in an open or closed network. In open networks, services at any community pharmacy is acceptable. In closed networks, only select community pharmacies can be used.

- In-house Network: The HMO facility generally houses and owns a pharmacy. Therefore, only members of the network receive pharmacy services.

- Mail Order Pharmacy Network: A managed care establishment owns and manages mail order pharmacies, which provide mail service to members for prescriptions. In addition, community pharmacies may fill prescriptions for members.

- Physician Dispensing Network: Medicines may be dispensed from the physician's office.

Plan Limitations
Plan limitations are used to control medication use and lower medication costs. In addition, plan limitations help determine plan savings.

Prescription Limitations
Prescription limitations establish maximal total drug quantities that may be distributed at a given time. For example, a daily limit is a 30-day supply for local pharmacies and a 90-day supply for postal order of drugs.

Drug Benefit Limitations
The drug benefit limitations express the total quantity can be dispensed at one time for a prescription. There should be a total number of prescriptions that can be dispensed to a customer per timeframe (usually monthly). There is a limited time frame for prescription refills, which is usually one year for drugs that do not contain a controlled substance.

Health Care Reimbursement Services
The Health Care Reimbursement Services contain four services as follows:

4 Types of Health Care Reimbursement Services	
Ambulatory care parenteral therapy	Codes for drugs on a list of health insurance continuation programs. This includes costs for reimbursement, professional fees, and facility fees.
Cognitive services	The pharmacist is given prescriptive power, drug administration, patient evaluation, therapy, prescribers' and other healthcare provider's involvement, education, reevaluation, and observation of patients. Based on the previous year's data, reimbursement is possible.
Community care	This involves drug prices, drug dispensing fees, observing, and record managing.
Long-term care	This is a predetermined daily rate determined by previous drug costs of the organization. Control of the formulary is paramount as regulatory establishments formulated a list of medicines they consider not necessary, determined by extreme adverse effects or insignificant results found.

Deductible
Before insurance coverage starts, a predetermined quantity of funds must be paid by the patient. Moreover, deductibles are not applicable to all prescriptions.

Types of Copayments
Among the three types of copayments, it is important to note that a patient is accountable for all prescription copayments and copays.

- Fixed copayment: when a prescription is filled, a prearranged dollar amount needs to be paid.

- Percentage copayment: a fixed percentage copayment is charged at the time the medication is dispensed, based on the total cost.

- Variable copayment: this is based on the type of medication dispensed. This is a variable or altered payment. Examples of these are generic drugs, preferential brand name drugs, non-preferential brand name drugs, etc.

Cost Containment

The process of cost containment involves these ten items:

- Limited pharmacy networks
- Postal-order and internet pharmacy
- Electronic request submission
- Greater member copayments
- Ranked copayments
- Formulary administration
- Prior approval
- Aggressive drug purchasing
- Benefit restrictions
- Compulsory generic replacement

Commercial Math Formulas

Cost	=	price of purchase + dispense cost
Discount	=	price of purchase × rate of discount
Discounted price	=	price of purchase − discount
Gross profit	=	price of selling item − price of purchase
Inventory turnover rate	=	annual dollar buying ÷ average inventory worth
Markup	=	price of selling item − price of purchase
Net profit	=	overall fee × desired percent gain
Overhead	=	total of all expenses
Profit	=	price of selling item − overall fee

Practice Questions

1. Conditions that may require authorization before prescription release to a patient would include which of the following?
   I. Generic medications available over brand name medications
   II. Medications that are too costly
   III. Age limit of drugs
   IV. Cosmetic drug use purposes only
   V. Non-life threatening drug use purposes only
   VI. Necessary prescribed drug by a doctor, but not covered by the insurance company
   a. I, II, IV, V
   b. II, III, VI
   c. I, IV, V, VI
   d. All of the above

2. Which formulary is defined as just a few medicines accessible in each medicinal group?
   a. Formulary Exception Process
   b. Open formulary
   c. Closed formulary
   d. Restricted formulary.

3. Which Medicare plan allows participants in Medicare Part A and B to get coverage via HMO or PPO for added services at a higher premium?
   a. Medicare Part A
   b. Medicare Part B
   c. Medicare Part D
   d. Medicare Advantage

4. Of the four types of health care reimbursement services, which involves drug prices, drug dispensing fees, observing, and record managing?
   a. Cognitive services
   b. Long-term care
   c. Ambulatory care parenteral therapy
   d. Community care

Answer Explanations

1. D: All of the conditions listed require authorization before prescription release to a patient.

2. C: Closed formularies allow access to just a few medicines for each medicinal group. In some cases, a whole group of medicines is not accessible.

3. D: Medicare advantage allows participants in Medicare Part A and B to get coverage via a HMO or PPO for additional services for an increased premium.

4. D: Community care involves drug prices, drug dispensing fees, observing and record managing.

Information System Usage and Application

Pharmacy-Related Computer Applications for Documenting the Dispensing of Prescriptions

Health Information Technology
Health Information Technology might impose significant risk to patient safety if not appropriately operated or monitored. Errors in technology may result in mistakes in drug labeling and medication information. If system updates are incomplete or inconsistent, patient safety might be compromised.

The Joint Commission Recommendations to Prevent Patient Harm when Implementing Health Information Technology
All standardized order sets and plans should be formulated, tried, and approved by the pharmacy and therapeutics (P&T) committee before making the system live. Technology should provide barriers to potentially harmful computerized physician order entry (CPOE) drug orders. Pharmacists must review and sign off on orders made outside of common procedures. For all electronic order sets, the pharmacy and therapeutic committee oversight and consent should be used.

Health Information Standards
Ensure the need for exchange of material in the healthcare establishment. Pharmacies need standards governing electronic communication with hospitals, doctor's offices, laboratories, radiology departments, patients, and caretakers. Moreover, for billing, reimbursing, administering, and delivering clinical purpose, it is vital to interconnect electronically.

Standard Development Organizations
For pharmacy services, the National Council for Prescription Drug Programs (NCPDP) cultivates and preserves standards for every stage in the development of prescribing. SCRIPT is an e-prescribing standard founded by NCPDP. The transfer of prescription data in the midst of pharmacies, prescribers, intermediates, and payers is managed by SCRIPT standards.

NCPDP Standards for Electronic Prescribing Procedure
Batch transaction standard
Billing unit standard
Financial information reporting standard
Formulary and benefit standard
Medicaid subrogation
Member enrollment standard
Payment reconciliation payment tape format
Pharmacy identification cards
Post-adjudication standard
Prescription transfer standard
Telecommunication standard
Universal claim form
Medication history standard

Pharmacist Services Technical Advisory Coalition
There are seven pharmacy organizations of the Pharmacist Services Technical Advisory Coalition listed below:

Pharmacist Services Technical Advisory Coalition (PSTAC)
American College of Clinical Pharmacy
Academy of Managed Care Pharmacy
American Pharmacists Association
American Society of Consultant Pharmacists
American Society of Health System Pharmacists
National Association of Chain Drug Stores
National Pharmacists Association

Pharmacy Informatics
Pharmacy informatics focuses on the use of information technology and medicine information to determine drug usage for patients. Drug orders are validated with other patient documents, and then made and dispensed with supreme quality, thereby preventing unnecessary risks. Since databases are connected with insurance companies, drug orders are authenticated against formulary information and contracts to certify proper usage and payment.

E-Prescribing
E-prescribing refers to a paperless system of prescription data for prescribers, pharmacies, and payers. E-Prescribing joins healthcare providers, patients, and agencies in real time, and forms a record of drug history and communication.

Electronic Health Care Records
Electronic data of patient healthcare is produced by one or more appointments in any care distribution environment. This information contains the patient's demographics, progress notes, medicines, vital signs, medical history, immunizations, laboratory information radiology reports, and progressive orders.

Computerized Physician Order Entry
The clinical information system allows a provider to enter an order for drugs, clinical laboratory tests, or radiology tests into the computer. Then the system transfers the orders to the appropriate department or person in order for the entire process to be carried out.

Telepharmacy
When a patient is unable to come to the pharmacy, the pharmacy may bring care to the patient. Real-time counseling is possible through video conferencing. Pharmacy services are provided through cost-effective techniques.

Technology and the Health Insurance Portability and Accountability Act (HIPAA)
HIPAA helps keep identifiable patient information confidential and protected. The Act allows medical records to be accessible to patients and their approved delegates only after written permission is granted. Technology used in the care of patients must comply with HIPAA, including electronic prescriber order entry. Patient data is transportable, moved between systems, and warehoused on the Internet with the appropriate protocol.

Documentation

In the documentation of medication-related dilemmas, coding systems are used. The documentation principles are as follows:

- Unique patient identification: When recording or retrieving data, unique identification is applied to each patient.

- Accuracy: Stored data and reports should be accurate and precise.

- Completeness: All recorded data should uphold legal, regulatory, organization policy, or other requisites. The minimum data required to finish the incident, surveillance, or intent should be reported.

- Timeliness: Documentation of healthcare is required during or directly after the encounter.

- Interoperability across documentation systems: Whether paper or electronic, approved practitioners should be granted permission to obtain, share, and report data from any system.

- Retrievability: Use of regulated titles, formats, templates, macros, terminology, abbreviations and coding should be activated, as should approved information searches, indexing, and mining.

- Authentication and accountability: Persons, instruments, and systems that will produce data and establish accountability for data's preciseness and timeliness should be identified.

- Auditability: Basic data elements are information fields, audit accessibility, and the Protected Health Information (PHI) disclosure, which should be examined by users. Users should be informed when errors, unacceptable changes, and potential security disruptions occur. The use of performance metrics should be encouraged.

- Confidentiality and security: Throughout the documentation process, all legislation, regulations, guidelines, and policies should be followed. Users should be mindful not to break the law through security breaches and confidentiality.

Ambulatory Pharmacy Computer Functions

A pharmacy database should contain the following:

- Drug file: Contains abbreviations, brand and generic name, price structure

- Physician file: Contains physician's phone number, address, Drug Enforcement Administration (DEA) number, National Provider Identifier (NPI)

- Clinical monitoring: Contains information regarding drug interactions, drug to food relations, drug to disease relations, drug to laboratory test relations

- Payer and insurance data

Each pharmacy should also have specific data for their patients and drugs entered into the system. This will allow such information to be transmitted to other systems or among providers and payers and helps keep up-to-date records. Patient information includes age, address, phone, sex, allergies, weight, height, diagnosis, insurance information, and information regarding the patient's medical needs and providers. Prescription processing information includes the patient's medical number, medication name, route, dose, route frequency, duration, and expiration date; the medication quantity and permissible refills, specific instructions or remarks, receipts, verification, label generation, price structure, etc. The information entered by technicians should be reviewed and verified by the pharmacist.

These systems also have management functions such as the ability to create reports, which can help assess and develop workflow. Possible reports include items such as distribution reports, financial reports, patterns of drug use, cost of drugs, performed jobs, etc.

Patient Monitoring Functions
Patient monitoring functions are identified as the clinical decision support system (CDSS).

Patient observing tasks involve examination of the following items:

- Therapeutic duplications: spots patients on medications in the same pharmacology therapy group.

- Drug to allergy interactions: uses the medical record to identify that a particular drug poses an allergy risk to a patient.

- Drug to drug interactions: identifies if multiple drugs taken together can cause problems.

- Drug to food interactions: alerts the patient that a drug taken with specific foods may cause a problem.

- Drug to disease interactions: involves medications that may exacerbate a patient's medical condition.

- Drug to laboratory test interactions: spots drug orders that may disrupt a specific laboratory test(s).

- Intravenous (IV) compatibilities: examines drug orders for possible interactions with IV usage.

Other Patient Monitoring Functions
In order not to exceed the ultimate dose, doses should be screened, particularly those that are known to cause adverse effects in pregnant or nursing patients. Patient populations like neonatal, pediatric, and geriatric should have specific dosing guidelines due to pharmacokinetics. For optimal care continuity, intervention documentation should be used.

Databases, Pharmacy Computer Applications, and Documentation Management

Inventory and Narcotic Control
Inventory and narcotic control record costs, purchase and usage, surplus, and outdated inventory. Borrowed medicines and supplies from other pharmacies should also be reported. When the Periodic Automatic Replenishment (PAR) level is reached, purchase orders need to be created. Purchase agreement records—including the minimum order for a drug, cost, payment policy, and return policy—should be kept on file.

Work Lists
Works lists are used with various pharmacy tasks. It is optional to print such lists daily or when needed. Work lists examples include items such as filling the unit dose cart, updating the cart fill, labelling, and updating the IV fill.

Work lists help determine the amount of each drug at a given period of time. Admission, discharge and transfer (ADT) notices, and drug administration records require document generation.

The Role of Automation

Automation refers to the use of machines to execute work. This includes storage, packaging, compounding, administering, and drug distributing. Automation has replaced intense labor jobs. The basic function of automation in pharmacies is to tally, package, and label dosage forms. Automation can also involve bar pricing, labelling, drug video imaging, barcoding, pricing, adjusting inventory, and documenting transactions.

Centralized and Decentralized Inpatient Automation Systems

Centralized automation systems are positioned in the central pharmacy and used to enhance manual filling unit dose carts. Advantages of these systems include the following: improved precision because they are based on barcoding, improved effectiveness for administrative tasks, reduced costs because items are purchased in bulk instead of unit doses, expiration dates can be track, inventory is better managed, and less time is needed to check technicians' work. The disadvantages are the cost of equipment, the cost of remodeling, and the inability to stock particular items like syringes or refrigerated goods.

Decentralized Automation Systems

Decentralized automation systems can be found in the patient care unit with stock drugs, supplies, and controlled substances on the unit floor. They have similar advantages and disadvantages as centralized systems, but they have the ability to stock items that are not possible with centralized systems.

Automation and Patient

The following features of automation have reduced the frequency of mistakes in pharmacies:

- Controls are clearly defined
- Barcoding or identification via electronics
- Drugs have limited and controlled accessibility
- Ability to capture dispensing and processing information
- Provision for drug use is available
- Labels are affixed and labeling machines are available
- The compromising of controls is designed to be a hindrance

National standards are not yet established for automation in pharmacies. As automation increases, more complex systems of distribution may occur; hence, added training for pharmacists and pharmacy technicians need to include:

- How to run a controlled pharmacy system
- How to recognize when there is a system failure
- How to safeguard patient safety when system failures occur
- How to fix errors and failures

Technologies Used in a Pharmacy

Automated dispensing systems contain methods to keep, administer, and charge stock drugs. For refrigerated medicines, some systems have the ability to refrigerate. Barcodes are used to detect a drug's dosage form and strength.

Barcode advantages	Barcode disadvantages
Because the barcode is portable, it can be used during prescription filling and examining at any location. The handheld device scans the NDC number on the barcode of the patient's label or receipt and confirms it with the scanned NDC number of the barcode on the stock medication container from which the prescription was filled.	Not all drugs are linked or barcoded to the dose.
	Not every medicine has a barcode, as there are numerous dosage types.
The nurse can scan the barcode on the patient's wristband before the giving a drug in a hospital. Directly after, the software compares information with the doctor's request to ensure the correct drug and dosage were dispensed to the right patient at the right time.	Installation of barcoding is costly.
This system establishes greater relations with the patient and care provider.	

Robotics

In pharmacy, robotics encompasses a centralized system of using barcode technology. It contains a chain of computers working cohesively. In this system of conveyors, robots are capable of choosing drugs from a patient's file, as well as putting the medicine in the right drawer for the given patient.

Automated Compounding Devices

Pumps that are run by computers are used to make ready IV admixtures (ingredients added to another substance) and total parenteral nutrition for adults and newborns. The device has pumps, which add the base solution, electrolytes, and nutrients. Also, some pumps can prefill syringes.

Paperless Charting

Without the use of paper, this system uses an electronic medical record for the patient.

Practice Questions

1. SCRIPT is an e-prescribing standard founded by which of the following?
    a. HIPAA
    b. PHI
    c. DEA
    d. National Council for Prescription Drug Programs

2. How many documentation principles for coding systems are used?
    a. 12
    b. 10
    c. 8
    d. 9

3. Patient monitoring functions are identified as the clinical decision support system (CDSS). Which of the following is NOT true?
    a. Therapeutic duplication, which spots patients on medication in the same pharmacology therapy group.
    b. Drug to allergy interactions, which identify that a particular drug may cause an allergic reaction in a given patient, given their medical history.
    c. Drug to disease interactions involve medicines that may exacerbate a patient's medical condition.
    d. Intravenous (IV) incompatibilities examine drug orders for medications that are not compatible with IV applications.

4. What system encompasses a centralized system in using barcode technology with conveyors capable of choosing drugs from a patient's file, as well as putting the medication in the right drawer for the patient?
    a. Automated pump system
    b. Automated dispensing systems
    c. Robots
    d. Automated tracking

Answer Explanations

1. D: The National Council for Prescription Drug Programs created the e-prescribing standard SCRIPT.

2. D: There are nine documentation principles used in coding systems. They are unique patient identification, accuracy, completeness, timeliness, interoperability across documentation systems, retrievability, authentication and accountability, auditability, and confidentiality and security.

3. D: Intravenous (IV) compatibilities examines drug orders for possible disruptions with IV applications.

4. C: Robots use barcode technology to choose drugs from a patient's file and can even put the medicine in the right drawer for the patient.

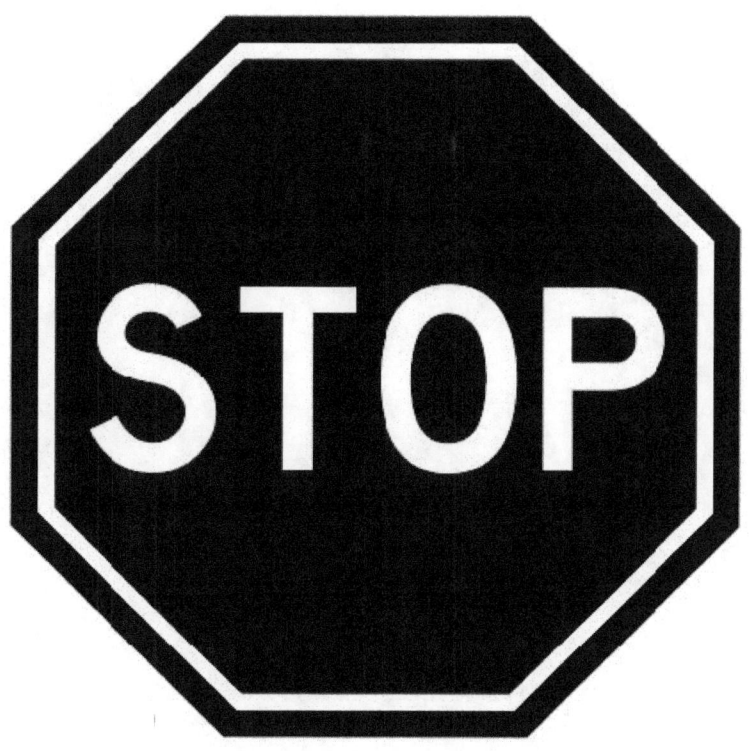

FREE Test Taking Tips DVD Offer

To help us better serve you, we have developed a Test Taking Tips DVD that we would like to give you for FREE. **This DVD covers world-class test taking tips that you can use to be even more successful when you are taking your test.**

All that we ask is that you email us your feedback about your study guide. Please let us know what you thought about it – whether that is good, bad or indifferent.

To get your **FREE Test Taking Tips DVD**, email freedvd@studyguideteam.com with "FREE DVD" in the subject line and the following information in the body of the email:

    a. The title of your study guide.

    b. Your product rating on a scale of 1-5, with 5 being the highest rating.

    c. Your feedback about the study guide. What did you think of it?

    d. Your full name and shipping address to send your free DVD.

If you have any questions or concerns, please don't hesitate to contact us at freedvd@studyguideteam.com.

Thanks again!